Also Available From the American Acad

Common Conditions

ADHD: What Every Parent Needs to Know

Allergies and Asthma: What Every Parent Needs to Know

The Big Book of Symptoms: A–Z Guide to Your Child's Health

Mama Doc Medicine: Finding Calm and Confidence in Parenting, Child Health, and Work-Life Balance

My Child Is Sick! Expert Advice for Managing Common Illnesses and Injuries

Sleep: What Every Parent Needs to Know

Waking Up Dry: A Guide to Help Children Overcome Bedwetting

Developmental, Behavioral, and Psychosocial Information

Autism Spectrum Disorders: What Every Parent Needs to Know

CyberSafe: Protecting and Empowering Kids in the Digital World of Texting, Gaming, and Social Media

Mental Health, Naturally: The Family Guide to Holistic Care for a Healthy Mind and Body

Newborns, Infants, and Toddlers

Caring for Your Baby and Young Child: Birth to Age 5*

Dad to Dad: Parenting Like a Pro

Guide to Toilet Training*

Heading Home With Your Newborn: From Birth to Reality

...enting Multiples From ...ancy Through the School Years

Retro Baby: Cut Back on All the Gear and Boost Your Baby's Development With More Than 100 Time-tested Activities

Your Baby's First Year*

Nutrition and Fitness

Food Fights: Winning the Nutritional Challenges of Parenthood Armed With Insight, Humor, and a Bottle of Ketchup

Nutrition: What Every Parent Needs to Know

A Parent's Guide to Childhood Obesity: A Road Map to Health

Sports Success R_X! Your Child's Prescription for the Best Experience

School-aged Children and Adolescents

Building Resilience in Children and Teens: Giving Kids Roots and Wings

Less Stress, More Success: A New Approach to Guiding Your Teen Through College Admissions and Beyond

Raising Kids to Thrive: Balancing Love With Expectations and Protection With Trust

For additional parenting resources, visit the HealthyChildren bookstore at **shop.aap.org/for-parents.**

*This book is also available in Spanish.

shop.aap.org

Baby Care Anywhere

Anywhere

A Quick Guide to Parenting On the Go

Ben Spitalnick, MD, MBA, FAAP, and
Keith Seibert, MD, MBA, FAAP

American Academy of Pediatrics
DEDICATED TO THE HEALTH OF ALL CHILDREN™

American Academy of Pediatrics Publishing Staff

Mark Grimes, *Director, Department of Publishing*

Kathryn Sparks, *Manager, Consumer Publishing*

Holly Kaminski, *Coordinator, Product Development*

Shannan Martin, *Publishing and Production Services Specialist*

Amanda Cozza, *Editorial Specialist*

Mary Lou White, *Director, Department of Marketing and Sales*

Mary Jo Reynolds, *Manager, Consumer Product Marketing*

About the American Academy of Pediatrics (AAP)
The AAP is an organization of 62,000 primary care pediatricians, pediatric medical subspecialists, and pediatric surgical specialists dedicated to the health, safety, and well-being of infants, children, adolescents, and young adults.

Published by the American Academy of Pediatrics
141 Northwest Point Blvd, Elk Grove Village, IL 60007-1019
847/434-4000
Fax: 847/434-8000
www.aap.org

Special discounts are available for bulk purchases of this book. E-mail our Special Sales Department at aapsales@aap.org for more information.

Front cover and book design by R. Scott Rattray
Cover photos by iStock

Baby Care Anywhere: A Quick Guide to Parenting On the Go was created by Ben Spitalnick, MD, MBA, FAAP, and Keith Seibert, MD, MBA, FAAP.

Library of Congress Control Number: 2014956224
ISBN: 978-1-58110-896-5
eBook: 978-1-58110-897-2
EPUB: 978-1-58110-912-2
Kindle: 978-1-58110-913-9

The recommendations in this publication do not indicate an exclusive course of treatment or serve as a standard of medical care. Variations, taking into account individual circumstances, may be appropriate.

Statements and opinions expressed are those of the authors and not necessarily those of the American Academy of Pediatrics.

Products and Web sites are mentioned for informational purposes only. Inclusion in this publication does not imply endorsement by the American Academy of Pediatrics. The American Academy of Pediatrics is not responsible for the content of the resources mentioned in this publication. Web site addresses are as current as possible but may change at any time.

Every effort is made to keep *Baby Care Anywhere: A Quick Guide to Parenting On the Go* consistent with the most recent advice and information available from the American Academy of Pediatrics.

This book has been developed by the American Academy of Pediatrics. The authors, editors, and contributors are expert authorities in the field of pediatrics. No commercial involvement of any kind has been solicited or accepted in the development of the content of this publication.

CB0085
9-362/0515

WHAT PEOPLE ARE SAYING

If there is only one book that parents read, this is it! Concise yet comprehensive; to the point and practical. An easy and very helpful read. Great book. Great gift.

Avril P. Beckford, MD, FAAP
Chief Pediatric Officer WellStar Health System
Past President, Georgia Chapter of the American Academy of Pediatrics

Baby Care Anywhere covers what you really need to know in quick and accessible bite-sized pieces! The perfect combination for busy parents!

Ari Brown, MD, FAAP
Pediatrician and author of *Baby 411* book series

Parents often lament that babies are born without operating instructions. Now, with the wealth of timely, important, and relevant tips provided by *Baby Care Anywhere,* they have them.

Paul A. Offit, MD, FAAP
Professor of Pediatrics, The Children's Hospital of Philadelphia

Here's the perfect "primer" for new parents! Clear, concise, and practical, the authors share their expertise in an accessible, friendly, and very informative style. This is the ideal book for parents to wrap their arms around the tasks and challenges of taking care of their infants and young children.

Steven P. Shelov, MD, MS, FAAP
Editor in Chief of *Caring for Your Baby and Young Child: Birth to Age 5*
Associate Dean, Undergraduate Medical Education
Winthrop University Hospital

CONTENTS

Part 3   Pediatric Checkups

Part 4 "What if My Baby Has...?" Top 10 Concerns Parents Bring to the Office

Part 5 A Doctor's Dozen: Top 12 Diagnoses Made in the Office

Part 6   **On the Go Info**

PREFACE

Welcome to parenthood—in the age of "information overload."

What started this project was a simple conversation over a cup of coffee. As the two of us compared similarities between our pediatric practices, we noticed a recurrent theme. We live in a world where advice is everywhere. It's in books, on the news, on the Internet, and in social media. Our friends e-mail, post, and blog advice. Parents (especially first-timers) have many of the same questions about their new baby, even though the answers are out there, in abundance.

Trying to find reliable advice while on the go can be tough. We have been there ourselves, not just as pediatricians but as parents. Recently, we were first-time parents too. More than once in our own homes, baby care advice we assumed as common knowledge was debated as inaccurate or not up-to-date. Our experiences drove home the point: parents need better access to quality, accurate information when they are out and about, away from their pediatrician's office or home.

The longer we practice, the more we hear the same questions, over and over. Should my baby *really* sleep on his back? When can we start using bug spray? Do vaccines cause autism? What can I use for cradle cap? (Yes. Two months. No. Adult dandruff shampoo.... But a lot more is ahead, so don't stop here.)

So we decided to create a book that's a field guide. We know your diaper bag follows your baby everywhere, so this book should be with you when baby questions come up. Think of it as the reference manual that should have come with your newborn.

Small enough to fit in your diaper bag, the book has a unique structure yet a range of topics, from picking a pediatrician you're comfortable with, to common questions parents ask, to top symptoms and diagnoses made in the office—all supported with advice from two board-certified pediatricians. Part 3, Pediatric Checkups, has individual pages for you to include questions you have and answers you receive from your well-child visits, as well as areas to write down all measurements and test results and how your child feels afterward. The book caps off with useful tips for traveling with a baby and offers a part for parents to keep track of must-pack items and information to remember while on the go.

We all want expert answers when an important health question comes up; now you have some at your fingertips wherever you go.

ACKNOWLEDGMENTS

When we started our various adventures together, the path was not toward creating a book. It was first toward improving our practices, then toward completing business school, and then toward developing medical devices. At some point, all the right influences fell into place, and we realized our experiences as pediatricians and parents might just make for a good read. But this project is a lot bigger than us two authors on the cover.

First, we have to thank Maria Lancaster. She is part mentor and part inspiration, and her support and encouragement have kept us on track for this book and many other endeavors (and, hopefully, more to come). If more meetings happened in coffee shops instead of offices, people in the world would have a greater number of good ideas.

Next, of course, we have to thank our respective pediatric practices. The running joke is that we never could have been so productive in our outside projects together if we were in the same medical practice. Thank you, SouthCoast Health and Pediatric Associates of Savannah, for giving us great places to practice, and, more importantly, helping us put our patients first.

The real spark to turn our idea into a publication has been our collaboration with the publishing team at the American Academy of Pediatrics (AAP). Mark Grimes took us under his wing, and Kathryn Sparks helped turn our "exam-room speak" into something that reads as clear as we wish we spoke. The AAP has helped us at every turn in our career, from residency, to practice, to leadership with the Georgia chapter. We are forever grateful to the AAP, and we hope we can continue to shape it as it shapes us.

Of course, we needed many reviewers to make sure we were going in the right direction. Thanks to Avril Beckford, MD, FAAP, and Bob Wiskind, MD, FAAP, for their expert advice, encouragement, and recommendations. Also, thanks to Ari Brown, MD, FAAP, for inspiration and for sage advice as well. Finally, thank you, Andrea Goto, for helping us find humor in writing and being gentle during our first-pass attempts to relearn grammar and vocabulary. And thank you to Stayce Koegler Photography for making us look better than real life.

Our families have been the source of unwavering support in this and many other projects and adventures (and misadventures). Dr Ben seems to always find one more new project, meeting, or committee to join, but without the encouragement and love of his wife, Alli, and daughter, Anna, such endeavors could not all happen (and he thanks his family for not throwing his laptop or iPad off a balcony when he's "busted" working on vacation). Dr Keith is grateful to his lovely wife, Heather, and his energetic daughters, Caroline and Camille, as they filled his world with joy (and princess music) during the writing of this book and were the inspiration for his work on it and every project.

Finally, but most importantly, none of these endeavors would happen, and this book certainly would not matter, without our patients. You have taught us much of what we know about life, pediatrics, and parenthood. We were told we would become better pediatricians when we had kids of our own (which has some truth to it). But the real lessons have come from daily interactions with you. Thanks for helping us write this book and for trusting us with your most precious gift.

Part 1

Welcome to the Doctor's Office

How to Pick Your Pediatrician

Several good pediatricians may practice in your area, and, as new parents, you will want to be sure you pick the "best" one. How do you decide which one is best for your baby?

We think the best way to pick your pediatrician is to start with the advice of your friends. You have friends and colleagues who share your values and who have children and thus see a pediatrician. Ask them. They will be honest. Ask if they are happy with their doctors and if they recommend them. If they are not happy with aspects of their doctors, ask why and who else they would consider if they switched. If you feel comfortable with your friend's opinion, see if your friend will you let you join him for one of his children's checkups. The doctor doesn't even need to know you're there as a prospective patient; pediatricians are used to parents bringing friends and family along to help them out. This way, you can see for yourself what the experience is like at the doctor's office. How friendly is the staff? What is the wait to see the doctor like? How well does the doctor relate to you? If the doctor turns out to be one you want to use, you can ask if she will take you on as a new patient. Even if the doctor has generally stopped taking new patients, some of us can't say no to a person in a face-to-face conversation.

Qualities to look for in a doctor really depend on your preferences. These may include

Is the Doctor Board Certified or Board Eligible?

In most states, doctors can practice without board certification, and you may not know if the doctor is board certified without asking. Usually a board-certified pediatrician will follow certain guidelines and principles of the American Academy of Pediatrics and must complete extensive continuing education requirements, whereas a non–board-certified pediatrician is not bound to such standards. If you see the letters *FAAP* (fellow of the American Academy of Pediatrics) after the doctor's name, she is board certified and has completed an intensive 3-year pediatric residency training program. But if you don't see them listed, ask anyway, as doctors don't always list all of their "letters."

Is the Doctor Full- or Part-time?

If the pediatric group has more than one office, does the doctor practice at the location you plan to use? Is the office open weekends and holidays? Who do you see if the doctor is away? Remember, you're not just picking your pediatrician for checkups; kids get sick 365 days a year, and you want to be able to reach your pediatricians or their partners for all care and spend as little time as possible in the emergency department or urgent care settings.

Does the Pediatric Group Have Electronic Medical Records?

Does the pediatric group have a Web site or social media page, such as Facebook, to alert you to office events, provide contact and doctor information, and list office hours? Does it have online access for appointment requests or to ask questions? As technology improves, patients and doctors have better access to medical information. Doctors who use electronic medical records can view your medical record after-hours from home or from multiple locations if they have more than one office. Along with such records, you may soon have direct online access through a "portal" where you can view laboratory results or immunizations, request appointments, or ask questions from the convenience of your mobile device or computer.

How to Make the Most of Your Pediatric Visit

Here are a few tips that you may find useful in making the most of your visit to your pediatrician.

✓ Complete Forms

If the pediatric group provides any paperwork that can be filled out prior to your visit, or prior to entering the examination room, go ahead and do so. That will give you more time to concentrate on your questions for the doctor and not be distracted by mounds of paperwork. Most of us are familiar with completing extensive forms the first time we visit a new doctor. Many pediatric check-ups require completing additional questionnaires that address development, exposure risks (such as to lead or tuberculosis), and safety questions. Many of these are standardized (ie, most doctors ask the same questions to be sure to screen for recommended problems), and they help identify areas that may need extra discussion or testing during your visit.

✓ Make Separate Appointments

Making separate appointments for each child may sound like a hassle or extra co-pay, but if you have multiple children who have different needs, we advise it. If your question is posed as, "While we are here with one child, we have a question about another child," your doctor may not be able to give your other children the time they deserve. The question about your other child may seem like a brief one at first. But to give it the attention you would expect, your pediatrician would likely require a complete history taking, physical examination, and chart review to ensure an accurate and thoughtful diagnosis and plan.

✓ Cut to the Point

Use the phrase, "The reason we are here today…" That will cut to the point of what your major concern is and help the conversation from getting lost to other smaller issues. If you have something important you want to discuss with your pediatrician, let the nurse know about it prior to him coming in. He is more likely to take time to listen to your concerns if he knows the reason you are there that day.

✓ Seek Assistance

If you have multiple children, finding a way to not bring them all to the doctor's office may be helpful. You will find yourself able to better focus on questions for the doctor if you are not busy keeping up with the other kids. An ideal situation would be to have a family member or babysitter stay with the other kids at home. Others find it helpful to bring a second adult along to the doctor's office. He can help with issues that may come up (such as another child needing to go to the bathroom). Or he may want to keep the other kids in the waiting room while you go back to the examination room with your child, which, again, gives you a better chance to focus on the visit.

✓ Don't Be Afraid to Ask

Nurses are gatekeepers to anything your doctor wants you to have at the end of the visit, such as formula, medical samples, or referral appointments. Do not hesitate to ask if they can help you, and know that they want to do an efficient job and can help your doctor take better care of your child.

✓ Get Familiar With Policies

Some office policies are not in the staff's control. For instance, privacy policies may prevent you from being able to send a family member or neighbor to pick up a prescription or medical records unless you call or write to authorize it. Likewise, if many parents are calling in for refills on the same day, plan on picking up prescriptions or documents the next day so that the staff has time to complete your request.

✓ Think Ahead

Before you leave, set up your child's next appointment. Whether it's a follow-up for an illness or your child's next checkup, staff behind the counter will know why you were there today and can schedule the appropriate next visit. This keeps you from having to remember to make the appointment later on, although some offices have call systems to remind you to set up a future appointment.

A notes section is included at the end of Part 1 where you can jot down important information from your child's initial visit, such as appointment days and times, phone numbers, and e-mail addresses.

Who's Who at Your Pediatrician's Office

Depending on the setting (such as a private practice, a university hospital, or a clinic), staff members may be somewhat different from those listed in this book, but generally you'll see the following ones in order of whom you may meet first:

✐ Front Desk Staff

Front desk employees handle a variety of tasks including, but not limited to, checking patients in, answering phone calls, and scheduling appointments. They are your gateway into the office and will try to make your waiting room experience as pleasant as possible.

✐ Clinical Staff

Clinical staff can include medical assistants, licensed practical (or vocational) nurses, and registered nurses. Each has a different level of training and experience and can help with various tasks, from measuring patients' vital signs, to taking part of the history, to answering medical phone calls.

✎ Your Pediatrician

Your pediatrician is an expert medical professional whose job it is to help keep your child healthy and on track developmentally. She is a doctor who oversees every aspect of your child's medical care, including evaluating symptoms and medical history, performing physical examinations, prescribing medication, and answering medical questions. Anything that happens in the office (eg, laboratory work, immunizations) is under her direction, even if she is not in the room when it is done. She will want to know how your experience is and will encourage you to ask any questions you have about your child's health.

✎ Other Pediatricians

Other doctors in the office have the same level of training as your doctor, may share nighttime or weekend responsibilities, and can help if your doctor is out of the office.

✐ Nurse Practitioners or Physician Assistants

Some pediatric groups include nurse practitioners or physician assistants. They are trained to independently handle common medical and well-child visit issues and should be in close contact with the doctor at your office about any complex issue. State law may require some percentage of their charts to be reviewed by the supervising doctor. These well-trained employees will also want to know about any compliment or concern you have.

✐ Office Manager

You most likely will never meet the office manager as part of your regular office visits, but she is who you would ask for if you have any concerns about the office or billing that needs extra attention. Depending on the type of pediatric group, she will be focused on ensuring that all people you encounter, and the office setting and rooms you find, are professional and efficient. She usually has the authority and responsibility to train, discipline, and reward front desk and nursing staff, so your feedback after your visit will always be welcome.

Pediatric Visit Notes

Pediatrician Office:

Pediatrician Name:

Staff Contact Names:

Office Address:

Office Phone Number:

Office Hours:

Notes :

_____

_____

_____

_____

_____

_____

_____

Pediatrician Office:

Pediatrician Name:

Staff Contact Names:

Office Address:

Office Phone Number:

Office Hours:

Notes:

_____

_____

_____

_____

_____

_____

_____

_____

_____

_____

_____

_____

_____

Pediatrician Office:

Pediatrician Name:

Staff Contact Names:

Office Address:

Office Phone Number:

Office Hours:

Notes:

_____

_____

_____

_____

_____

_____

_____

_____

_____

_____

_____

_____

_____

Future Appointments

Day: Time:
Office Address:

_____

_____

_____

Day: Time:
Office Address:

_____

_____

_____

Day: Time:
Office Address:

_____

_____

_____

Part 2

Frequent Questions Drs Ben and Keith Receive

What Should We Buy for Our Baby?

The number of items you could buy for your baby has no limit. A quick search online reveals countless baby items that await your consideration. When we brought our own babies home, we bought baby products that our patients' families recommended. Based on what we found useful, here are some important ones you *should* buy, and we'll leave all the optional cute ones up to you.

✓ Baby Monitors

Three categories of baby monitors are commercially available. In order of cost and complexity, these include sound-only monitors, video/sound monitors, and those that monitor baby movements. None are necessary but often give parents a sense of reassurance by providing some idea of what is going on in the next room.

 This book does not include medical apnea monitors, which are doctor prescribed and used rarely for medical conditions such as extreme prematurity.

Sound-Only Monitor

Many parents are reassured by a simple auditory monitor that allows them to hear if their baby is crying. If you are using an intercom type for just sound, it may have settings for different frequencies. Find one that has the least static or other noises to be sure you don't pick up sounds besides your own baby. Also, make sure it is positioned outside the crib. If you place it inside the crib, you may pick up the rustle of a mattress or diaper from your baby's movement, and this can sound like a loud, scary emergency is happening, instead of typical sleeping movement.

Video/Sound Monitor

Video/sound monitors are widely available and vary by technical abilities and cost. Most sit on a bookshelf or other stationary object and are positioned in a way that can provide a view of your sleeping baby. Some come with a corresponding handheld viewing screen, and others can be hooked into your home wireless network to be streamed to your cellphone, television, or tablet. Many have night vision functionality so you can see your baby even when all the lights are off. If you are using a video monitor, be sure to set it up so that it shows most of your baby's mattress. Otherwise, he's likely to roll just out of view, which defeats the purpose.

Movement-Monitoring Device

As technology improves, new movement-monitoring devices are available for purchase. Some attempt to monitor your baby's

Check Out Receipt

Laurel County Public Library

Thursday, August 3, 2017 3:31:02 PM

Title: Baby care anywhere : a quick guide to par
enting on the go
Due: 08/24/2017

Title: Help! i'm a dad : all a new dad needs to
know about the difficult first few months.
Due: 08/24/2017

Books, audiobooks, and CDs now have a 21 day
checkout period!
DVDs have a 7 day checkout period.
Fines begin to accumulate on days 22 and 8,
respectively.

Thank You!

breathing by detecting movement on the mattress. Others are wearable devices that try to accomplish the same purpose. These look appealing to new parents wanting to monitor their baby as closely as possible, but use can lead to a false sense of security. None of these devices has shown to help prevent the occurrence of sudden infant death syndrome (see What Is SIDS? on page 78).

✓ Breast Pump

If you plan to breastfeed your baby, you'll likely want to invest in a breast pump to help store breast (human) milk when you can. We suggest you try out the hospital version and talk to a lactation consultant before spending several hundred dollars on this item, as you'll understand the different brands and features before making a purchase. Most parents find the electric pump to be a lot more successful than the hand pump, as it is often easier to use and yields a larger amount of pumped milk.

✓ Clothing

Baby clothing is often sized for the smallest baby at that age. For example, 6-month-old clothing is designed for a small 6-month-old baby, meaning many 6-month-olds tend to fit in "older" baby clothing. Because of this, don't overbuy for any particular season, as your baby may grow out of that size clothing before the end of the season.

Especially in early infancy, your baby will often wear the same outfit several times, and you may be so exhausted that you won't even notice. Many parents want a few nice outfits for those special photographs and social media posts, but, in general, the best baby outfits are those easiest to use, especially the kind that don't require multiple snaps, buttons, or entire clothing removal for every diaper change and that allow for comfort and free movement.

✓ Diapers

At any baby shower, ask for as many cloth or disposable diapers as you can get. They will be needed! Try to get a wide variety of sizes, as you will be amazed at how quickly your baby grows out of newborn diapers and graduates to size one. Babies grow at different speeds, so the size your baby needs may not match the size on the box. Also, consider subscribing to a cloth diaper service or an online mass-purchasing program to keep your costs down and order as needed.

With disposable diapers, don't be surprised if one brand fits better than another. In Dr Keith's experience with his own children, one did great with a national brand, while the next had sensitive skin and did better when he tried cloth diapers.

Consider the disposal of diapers and wipes as well. Several companies make specialized diaper-disposal trash cans. You may know these already; they take the diaper (and wipes) and spin them into a small plastic bag to seal off the smell. What you have left will look like a sausage-link diaper chain. Diaper-disposal trash cans can be useful if you want to have a trash can for diapers right near your changing station, but even the best ones start to smell after a while. If you live in a house with a garage, or easy access to an outside trash can, skip this item and just take the diapers outside.

Cloth diapers are useful and greener, but in the early days you might go through 10 to 15 diapers in a day, so be ready to rinse the diaper out and do the laundry more often than you ever imagined. Many versions have a disposable inner liner to try to reduce the mess.

✓ Fingernail File or Clippers

Many parents worry about the right way to trim their new-born's fingernails. Nails grow quickly and are often sharp right from birth, and, if you do nothing, your newborn is certain to accidentally scratch her face or you. You will only have so much success in keeping mittens (or socks) on her hands. Some parents prefer to file the nails down, although this takes time. Infant fingernail clippers are safe to use. You should be able to slide the clipper just along the fingernail and gently pull the skin back from the fingertip. If you are worried, no harm in trimming a little and going back for more later. You may even find success if you try this while your baby is sleeping.

✓ Starter Kit

Many parents find it helpful to create a kit to store their baby-related health items. This helps keep everything in one place so you (or other caregivers such as grandparents) can find everything specific to your baby. It also makes grabbing everything to be packed easier if you and your baby are on the go. You should store it somewhere convenient to you but somewhere separate from the rest of your family's medicines or health items to avoid confusion. If you are making a starter kit, here are items we think you should include.

- ☐ Acetaminophen (See Fever on page 163 prior to use.)
- ☐ Baby shampoo
- ☐ Gas relief drops
- ☐ Medicine dropper
- ☐ Nail file
- ☐ Nasal bulb
- ☐ Nasal saline drops
- ☐ Petroleum jelly
- ☐ Safety fingernail clippers
- ☐ Thermometer
- ☐ Zinc oxide–based diaper cream

✓ Strollers

Strollers are an essential tool for families on the go and come in several styles. The type you buy will vary on your expected use, and you may end up with more than one. Different types to consider include

Jogging Strollers

Jogging strollers are rugged and sporty and great for taking your baby with you while you get some exercise. They come in 3- and 4-wheel models. These are generally not for use with babies younger than 6 months.

Multiples Strollers

Multiples strollers? Yes, they make strollers to accommodate 2 or 3 babies at the same time. These are designed either side by side or "limousine" style (one behind the other).

Seat Carriers

Seat carriers are sold to complement your baby's car seat; simply release the car seat from your car and pop it into the seat carrier. This is convenient in the first few months, especially if your baby is sleeping and you don't want to wake him. The downside, however, is that once your baby outgrows the car seat, the matching seat carrier has no use.

Traditional Strollers

Traditional strollers have the largest variety in size, style, and cost. Most are for older babies and children, but some can hold younger babies by converting into a bassinet-type carriage. These are usually more lightweight than the two strollers already mentioned. But they are not used with a car seat; thus, transferring baby from car seat to stroller is a little more work.

Travel Systems

Travel systems are similar to seat carriers but have the ability to be used as a traditional stroller seat when your baby outgrows his car seat. These are usually sold with a matching car seat and have the same advantages as the seat carrier but are usually bulkier and more expensive.

Regardless of which you choose, safety and installation of a seat/stroller vary based on product and type. Always refer to the manufacturer's guide to ensure proper installation and correct use. Check your community resources. Some communities have a "safety village," or the local fire department is sometimes set up to do car seat checks for safety and installation.

✓ Swaddle Blanket

Swaddling a baby can be an effective way to help a baby sleep. Many infant blankets can be used to swaddle, but some are designed to specifically make swaddling easier. We don't mention brand names, but in Dr Ben's experience with his own daughter, a swaddle blanket was just the miracle he and his wife needed for all to get a little more sleep. If you use a swaddle blanket, practice safe sleep techniques: make sure your baby is still sleeping on his back (faceup), no loose blankets are in the crib, and he is not too hot.

How Do I Give My Baby a Bath?

One of the first experiences you may witness in the hospital following the birth of your baby is her first bath. During your baby's first years, her bath will be quality bonding time for your family, so here are some quick tips.

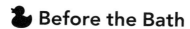 Before the Bath

Temperature

Check water temperature early and often. Make sure your hot water heater is set to a maximum temperature of 120°F (49°C) to minimize risk of burns. Mix in warm and cool water, and test the temperature on a sensitive part of your body to gauge whether it's too hot for your baby.

Supplies

Keep all your supplies handy, including soap, washcloths, basins, towels, and any wraps you plan on using for your baby afterward.

🦆 During the Bath

Sponge Bath

Before the umbilical cord stump falls off and the base of the umbilicus (belly button) heals, plan on sponge baths. This means placing your baby in a safe and supervised position on a towel or a changing table and rinsing her body with a warm wet washcloth. No soap is needed for the face in her first week; for the rest of her body, only use a mild soap and washcloth. Her skin oils are important, and over-washing can contribute to dry skin. It's often hard to wash and rinse in skin folds, such as under the neck and in the thighs. Be sure to pay extra attention to do a thorough job in these areas. The first few times you bathe your baby, an extra set of hands (such as from a spouse or grandparent) will be helpful.

Soap-and-Water Bath

Babies do not need much soap, and over-washing is usually more of a problem than under-washing. Bathing with soap 2 to 3 times per week is often sufficient during the first year of life. Many parents find it helpful to have an extra towel ready in case they need to pick up their baby in the middle of a bath. Check water temperature often during the bath.

Shampooing the scalp once or twice per week is usually plenty, and using a shampoo with selenium sulfide (leave it on for 20 to 30 seconds, rinse thoroughly, and avoid the baby's eyes) can help alleviate scaly scalp rashes such as cradle cap (see Diagnosis: Cradle Cap on page 187). Ask your doctor first if you have questions about any baby rashes.

After the Bath

Your baby is sensitive to the cold, so place her in the water immediately after she is undressed, and pat her dry immediately after taking her out of the bath.

After you pat your baby dry, applying a gentle fragrance-free hypoallergenic baby lotion can help prevent overly dry skin.

If you need to receive a phone call, answer the door, or perform any task, bring your baby. Never leave her alone, even for a second.

Is This a Birthmark or a Rash?

New parents may have questions about spots on their baby's skin: Are the spots birthmarks? A new baby rash? Will it go away? Will it grow or shrink? Does it need treatment? Some parents may be surprised to know that not all birthmarks are present the day a baby is born; some can become apparent over the first few weeks or months of life. The following is a list of birthmarks and baby rashes we are asked about, starting with the most common.

Stork Bites and Angel Kisses

What Are These?

Stork bites are flat, red/pink, and smooth and are also known as salmon patches. They often appear as a cluster just above the back of the neck, thus the name stork bites, because this is where the stork would pick a baby up if that were, in fact, how babies were delivered (PS it isn't). These often go unnoticed (they can be mild and sometimes covered by hair on the back of the head) and occur in one-third of babies. When they appear on the forehead and are thus more noticeable, they're given the nickname "angel kisses." Angel kisses can appear as a V-shape on the forehead, small pink spots on the upper eyelids, or small dots on the lower forehead.

Will They Go Away?

Stork bites and angel kisses almost always go away with time, and nothing needs to be done to rid of them.

Strawberry Hemangiomas

What Are These?

Hemangiomas are collections of capillaries (small blood vessels) that often are unnoticeable at birth but start to grow over the first few weeks of life. They start off as flat and pink, but, over a few weeks, turn bright red and raised, and the top can have a "cauliflower" or "strawberry" texture. These often concern parents because of their rate of growth in a baby from 2 to 4 months of age.

How Long Do They Last?

A strawberry hemangioma will occur in 10% of babies by 2 months old; however, most appear by 2 to 3 weeks. They typically grow through infancy, stop, and slowly go away over the next 1 or 2 years. Eventually, most strawberry hemangiomas completely go away without any residual scar or coloration, or treatment, needed. The recommendation for most hemangiomas is to tell your doctor so both of you can simply keep an eye on its development. Some rare large ones may require treatment because they will not improve on their own, but your doctor will be able to determine if this is necessary.

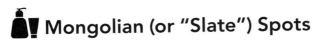 Mongolian (or "Slate") Spots

What Do They Look Like?

When we first started training, mongolian spots referred to bluish spots on the lower back and buttocks, which often look like a large bruise. But as we become more politically correct, the term is being replaced by "slate" spots. Some people mistake these marks for a bruise. Bruises appear bluish at first and, over 1 or 2 days, change to green and yellow as the bruise starts to fade. Slate spots have a consistent bluish color throughout that does not change.

Will They Go Away?

Slate spots are more common in darker-skinned babies and often fade over the first few months of life, but they may persist, often for a few years and in some cases for life. Either way, these spots do not pose any health risks to your baby and do not require treatment.

Erythema Toxicum

While erythema toxicum has a scary-sounding name, the flea-bite-looking spots it consists of appear around the time of birth and usually fade in the first few weeks of life. They often start on the face and trunk (ie, chest, belly, and back) and can spread to the arms and legs. Many studies have confirmed that they are just common accumulations of little white blood cells, called eosinophils, which are harmless and need no treatment.

Pustular Melanosis

Pustular melanosis can look like little scaling circles, brown circular spots, or, sometimes, little pimply bumps. If you ever see fluid-filled blisters with worsening redness, tell your pediatrician (because this could be a sign of infection), but small scaling spots or light brown spots are typical.

What Should I Know About Breastfeeding or Formula Feeding?

Many studies have shown that breastfeeding holds long-lasting benefits for both mothers and babies. If you plan to breastfeed your baby, this chapter may help answer some of your questions.

What Are the Benefits of Breastfeeding?

In general, the longer you breastfeed, the better for you and your baby.

- Breastfeeding helps create the special bond between mother and baby.
- Breast milk provides special nutrients for babies that reduce rates of food allergy, colic, and eczema and may improve their development later on.

- Breast milk is almost always available, free, and ready to feed and adapts to meet your baby's changing needs as he grows.
- Breastfeeding helps a mother's hormones rebalance, helps her lose weight by burning additional calories, helps keep iron in her body by delaying return of the menstrual cycle, and reduces risk of ovarian and breast cancers.

How Soon After Birth Does a Baby Start to Breastfeed?

Talk with your delivery team about helping you place your baby on your breast as soon after delivery as possible (called "skin to skin" placement). This helps your baby handle the stress of delivery and helps your body finish the birthing process.

How Do I Help My Baby Latch On and Find the Best Position?

When holding your baby and supporting her head and neck with one hand, use your free hand to guide your breast toward her mouth. Gently touch your nipple to her lower lip, which prompts her reflexes to open her mouth. Be sure that she takes most of your areola in her mouth, and remember that both her nose and chin should be touching your breast. A good latch-on should satisfy your baby more easily, stimulate your body to make more milk, and minimize any pain or discomfort you may be having. A lactation consultant should be available to you at the hospital for further assistance.

Common breastfeeding positions include

- **Cradle hold.** Hold your baby across your body as you support her head, back, and bottom.
- **Football hold.** Hold your baby under one arm, with your arm supporting her body and your hand supporting her head. This position is great if you have had a cesarean delivery (commonly referred to as a C-section), as it keeps your baby off of your incision.
- **Reclining position.** Your baby lies next to you, and your bed supports her weight as she feeds.

 ## How Often and for How Long Does a Baby Breastfeed? How Much Milk Does a Baby Need?

The frequency and timing of breastfeeding can be all over the map. Babies breastfeed every 1 to 3 hours (anywhere from 8 to 12 times per day) or more during the first few weeks of life, and they only need a small amount—as few as 1 to 2 tablespoons—of the thick early milk (known as colostrum) during their first few days. This amount increases with your baby's growth. Generally, most nutrition comes in the first 20 to 30 minutes on each breast, so feeding more than 40 minutes total (after the high-fat milk at the end of the feeding, the so-called hind milk) is probably wearing your baby out and irritating your breasts, so talk with your lactation consultant about this.

Episodes of "cluster feeding"—during which a baby continually feeds, falls asleep, wakes to feed after a few minutes, and keeps up this cycle for a few hours—can be exhausting but is an expected part of his hunger drive and the signal to your body to make more milk. Likewise, "growth spurts" occur every few weeks and include several days of increased appetite. Concerns regarding whether a baby is feeding enough are best addressed with a simple weight check at your pediatrician's office.

How Do I Know When My Milk Has Come In?

Many women whose milk has come in feel their breasts become engorged, or swollen; often feel tingling in their nipples; see milk leaking from their breasts or their baby's mouth; and can hear their baby swallowing milk during feedings.

What Do I Do if I Do Not Feel My Breastfeeding Is Going Well?

Your pediatrician and your lactation consultant are trained to help you with any difficulties you may be having with breastfeeding, so call them as soon as you see the need.

How Can I Continue to Make Milk When I'm On the Go or Back at Work?

Many women are able to successfully express milk, by hand or with an electric pump, during their return to work or when they need to be away from their baby. Numerous bags for freezing and storage exist and can keep your milk ready until you return to your baby. Babies can learn to accept breast milk from a bottle, so talk with your pediatrician or lactation consultant about how to work this into your routine.

What's My Baby's Father's Role in Breastfeeding?

By cuddling a fed baby, by learning to understand the baby's cues and provide for her needs, and by supporting and encouraging a breastfeeding mother, a father can bond with his baby and really help in the process of feeding.

Breastfeed Until What Age?

The American Academy of Pediatrics and World Health Organization suggest mothers exclusively breastfeed until their babies are 6 months old; continue breastfeeding, and add complementary solid foods, until 1 year; and breastfeed after that as long as mother and baby desire. The American Academy of Pediatrics notes that studies show no increase in food allergies when complementary solid foods are started as early as 4 months, so parents should watch their baby, talk with their pediatrician, and come to their own decision. Finally, remember that breastfeeding does not have to be an all-or-none choice. If you're making some breast milk, you can breastfeed your baby some of the time, or express breast milk (by hand or pump) and feed it to your baby, in addition to formula. You can add it directly to formula, but remember that the mixture should be fed to your baby at that time and not stored until later.

Some experts recommend weaning at 1 year, as a baby is more flexible than he might be later on. Remember that patience and understanding is important, as a baby may not be ready to wean at this point or you may want to continue breastfeeding longer than this. Regardless of when you choose to wean, you may want to help your baby learn to take a bottle of pumped breast milk during his infancy, as this may make it easier to wean later on.

What Are My Options if We Use Formula?

If formula is your choice, several nutritious brands are available, all of which are regulated by the US Food and Drug Administration and provide similar calories, protein, and nutrients. But each has its own advantages. While each may differ in cost and availability, you can ask your pediatrician about her recommendation. Remember, breast milk is the gold standard, so the goal of formula is to get as close to breast milk as possible. While many formulas are on grocery store shelves, all can be broken down into a few main categories, which are listed below in order of what is most commonly recommended, and usual cost. Keep in mind, like many things, more expensive does not always mean what is best for your baby.

- **Standard (milk-based) formulas** are tolerated by most babies and are a good first choice when not breastfeeding.
- **Hydrolyzed whey-protein formulas** are made from only some of the proteins in whole cow's milk and may give a slightly lower risk of eczema later in infancy.
- **Formulas based on soy proteins,** or those that are lactose reduced/lactose free, are an option for the baby who struggles with standard formulas.
- **Predigested or hydrolyzed formulas,** ranging from partially to completely broken down, are good options for especially colicky babies with food allergies. We recommend checking with your doctor before switching formulas.

What if My Baby Seems Gassy or Fussy While Feeding?

Remember, all babies will be gassy from time to time (see Diagnosis: Colic on page 184), even when they are on the best formula for them. Gas, alone, is not a reason to change your diet while breastfeeding or to change formulas. Also, if you switch formulas, it can take as long as several days to see benefits or other changes.

 ## If I Choose to Bottle-feed My Baby, Which Bottle and Nipple Should I Use?

Various bottles and different sizes and styles of nipples are available. Babies who are breastfeeding as well as bottle-feeding may do well on a slower-flow nipple, as they may not be used to quickly flowing milk. You will see age recommendations for different bottles and nipples, and promises of easy feedings and less gas, but every baby is different, so start with one slowly, and experiment from there.

Baby Foods: When and How Do We Start Solid Foods?

At first attempt when starting solid foods, introduce a new food every 3 days or so to allow time to see if your baby is going to have a reaction or digestive problem. This may include upset tummy symptoms, such as vomiting or diarrhea, or a skin symptom, such as a blotchy rash. Most of these get better with time, but it's useful to know what is sensitive to your baby's system. If a symptom is mild (such as a loose stool or increased gas), you can avoid the food for a few weeks and reintroduce it to see if it has the same result. If a rash develops over her body, talk with your pediatrician before giving that food again (and take a picture of the rash if you can't see your pediatrician quickly so that he can see what it looked like).

What Do the Food Stages Really Mean?

Here's a helpful guide to what the food stages really mean.

- **Stage 1** foods are pureed to a thin mixture, and each jar contains 2 ounces of food.
- **Stage 2** foods are a little thicker, and each jar contains 4 ounces of food.
- **Stage 3** foods have some chunks of solid food, and each jar contains 6 ounces of food.

When you first start feeding your baby, she'll likely only be able to take a few teaspoons, and even those will involve a lot of spitting and sputtering. Slow down, have fun, and don't worry if she's not eating much yet. In fact, she might just take half a stage 1 jar. At the beginning, eating is about how textures feel in the mouth and improving tongue/swallow coordination. It's not really about taste, and within a few days' time, she'll be eating a whole stage 1 jar (2 ounces) without much trouble.

How Long Do Babies Last in Each Stage?

In terms of schedule, most babies stay on stage 1 jars—fed twice a day (usually morning and evening), working through vegetables, then fruits—for about 2 months (from 4 until 6 months of age for early starters, from 6 until 7 or 8 months for the start-at-6-months camp). This usually doesn't affect their total formula or breast milk intake. They then move to stage 2 foods, also spend a couple months working through the various options, and usually feed 3 times a day. At this point, their breast milk or formula intake noticeably starts to decrease. Finally, usually around 9 to 10 months, babies start on stage 3 foods 3 times a day and learn to swallow little bits of food as they get ready for the switch to table foods by 1 year. They may also be ready to handle little finger foods, such as puffs and teething crackers designed and made for babies at this age, as snacks between meals. Milk intake often drops down to 20 to 24 ounces per day.

What Is the Best Feeding Schedule?

There are as many different feeding regimens as there are parents. Most pediatricians try to steer away from a detailed feeding schedule because every baby is different and not all do well with the same foods in the same order. Don't stress too much if you find out your friends' babies are following a different food order than your baby (eg, vegetables before or after starting fruits, green colors before or after orange ones). There's no correct order of serving foods.

Can We Make Our Own Baby Foods?

Feel free to make your own baby foods! Although most commercially prepared baby foods are safe and nutritious, you can certainly make your own baby foods from fresh fruits and vegetables. Be sure to check the consistency of typical stage 1 and stage 2 baby foods first to get an idea of how thick or thin the food should be. Recipes are online, and they shouldn't call for much more than the fruit or vegetable, a little olive oil or water, and minimal flavorings. A good rule of thumb is to see what is already on shelves in the baby food section of your grocery store.

Should We Avoid Any Foods Because of Possible Allergies?

Some doctors advise to delay giving nuts, peanut butter, fish, shellfish, and eggs until a child is 1 year old because of concern for allergic reactions, especially if you have a family history of food allergies; however, there is no convincing evidence that doing so will determine whether your baby may be allergic to them. Some recommend introducing one new food at a time to check for reactions. Talk with your doctor about this if you have questions or see signs of allergies, such as swelling, rash, hives, and diarrhea, after your baby eats specific foods.

Can My Baby Have Honey?

Do not give raw honey to your baby during the first year. If eaten, she is at risk of severe bacterial infection.

When Do We Start to Offer Meat?

Meats can be pureed and be part of stage 2 foods (and many pre-prepared jars include meats), and some people even start these with stage 1 foods. If you are making your own baby food, you can puree basic meats (ie, beef, pork, chicken) to the same consistency as other baby foods.

Can My Baby Feed Herself Solid (Finger) Foods?

Your baby may learn to feed herself a few soft foods when she is able to sit up in a high chair, reach for her food, and bring it to her mouth. As the American Academy of Pediatrics recommends, minimize the risk for choking by only giving your baby soft foods that are easy to swallow and cut into small pieces. Some parents try yogurt melts, bits of banana, dissolved wafer-type cookies or crackers, scrambled eggs, or well-cooked and diced pasta, chicken, and vegetables.

How Do I Baby-Proof My Home?

Poison Help: 1-800-222-1222

Preparing your home to be a safe place for your new baby should start from day one. If you wait until he is active and moving, you are behind the action. *Be on the lookout!* It is very common for your baby or toddler to be injured by things he never showed interest in before.

When looking to baby-proof your home, a good way to start is on your hands and knees. By that, we mean you should crawl around and see what you hit your head on (sounds silly but can be eye-opening!).

Sharp corners should be covered up, especially on fireplaces and end tables. Some parents will remove the coffee table from the living room for a few months during the early walking period.

Stairs should be blocked off (at top and bottom if your child spends time in both places).

Cabinets and drawers can be and should be safety locked.

Infant walkers can be a source of injury when they overturn or lead to falls, especially down stairs. Most pediatricians do not recommend walkers because of these injuries.

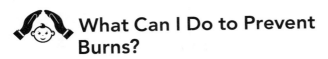 What Can I Do to Prevent Burns?

Burns are an all-too-common occurrence in babies and can come from several sources, including hot water, hot surfaces, and fireplaces.

- Your water heater should have a temperature set at 120°F (49°C) or lower to prevent burns from hot water.
- Burns from contact with hot surfaces (such as the stove in the kitchen or clothing or hair-care irons) are best prevented by close supervision and gates, closed doors, or barriers to prevent access.
- When heating foods in the microwave, be aware that "hot spots" within the bottle or food can develop, causing mouth burns even if the bottle or bowl does not feel too hot.

Fire and smoke alarms, as well as carbon monoxide detectors, can help identify these important dangers in time to extinguish them or safely leave the home.

Likewise, **fireplaces** should have a solid barrier, not just a mesh wire, to keep your kids away from any part of the fire. Call 911 if you need any help. **Radon** is a colorless, odorless gas released by natural uranium deposits in the ground and one cause of lung cancer. Simple home detectors can detect its presence.

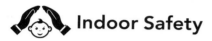 Indoor Safety

All **electrical outlets** should be covered, and small hard-to-remove covers are available at all large department stores. If you are aggressive about baby-proofing, the outlets can be changed out to a fancier kind with baby-proofing features built in. Power cords should also be covered and protected from curious hands.

A child can use an electric cord to pull things down and get hurt from **falling objects** (especially televisions or other desktop appliances) or can be injured while teething and chewing on a power cord.

Some common **houseplants** can be dangerous if their leaves, berries, or stems are ingested. Call Poison Help at 1-800-222-1222 for a list of plants that should be avoided.

Chemical and Medication Safety

Latches and locks can prevent access to dangerous cleaning chemicals or home pesticides under the kitchen sink or in the bathroom, such as drain cleaners or bleach. Children look at things differently than adults do, and you will be amazed at how edible cleaning supplies look to a kid (such as the refreshing blue shimmer of glass cleaner or the shiny candy-like appearance of dishwasher pods). Drawers that contain medication need to be outfitted with a variety of locks and latches that can protect toddlers from these exposures. Better yet, move medication out of drawers into higher places such as cabinets. **Medications** often include baby-resistant packaging, although these aren't always effective, so focus on locking them away and keeping them out of reach.

How Do I Keep My Baby Safe Outside?

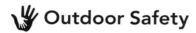 Outdoor Safety

When Should I Use Sunscreen?

Protection from the sun is easily overlooked in young infants. Sunscreen is safe to start using on small areas of exposed skin as young as 4 to 6 months of age and more liberally after 6 months. It should be applied at least 30 minutes before going into the sun and have both UVA and UVB protection (the label should say "broad spectrum"). And, yes, even on a cloudy day an infant can experience the effects of sun exposure, so pick sunscreen with a sun protection factor (SPF) of at least 15. Most pediatricians recommend an SPF of at least 30. For an SPF of greater than 30, the increased protection, as indicated by the higher rating number, is minimal. Most people put on too little sunscreen, so apply a generous amount. It should be reapplied throughout the day about every 2 hours, especially if time is spent in the water, sweating, or toweling off. For the most exposed areas of skin (eg, nose, cheeks, ears, shoulders), consider a sunscreen with zinc oxide or titanium dioxide. These ones generally don't fully rub in, and stay visible, and now come in colors your child may find fun.

Should I Use Bug Spray or Insect Repellant to Prevent Bites?

Bug repellant is also important for outings, especially time spent outdoors in mornings and evenings. Bug spray should not be used on babies younger than 2 months; for older than 2 months, it can, but check with your pediatrician if you have concerns. DEET is the most common active ingredient in bug sprays, and the concentration will vary among different products. DEET concentration is found on the front label of most commercially available insect repellant, written out as "N,N-diethyl-meta-toluamide." Studies show that DEET concentration is related to how long protection will last; 10% should last about 2 hours, and 24% should last about 5 hours. Concentrations greater than 30%, however, have not shown much extended benefit and are not recommended for children. DEET insect products should be applied no more than once a day.

Some parents want to try DEET-free or "natural" alternatives, and there are some out there that may be effective (generally not as effective as DEET, however). These include products made from oils of citronella, cedar, eucalyptus, or soybean plants. Options that are generally not effective, however, include oral garlic, "ultrasonic" devices that are supposed to emit ultrasound noises, and wristbands soaked in chemicals. While backyard bug zappers may appear to be doing a good job, they may actually attract more bugs to your yard than they kill. Also, for young infants, a mosquito net securely attached to a stroller is a great way to go for walks and get outdoors.

The American Academy of Pediatrics recommends avoiding the combination of sunscreen and DEET products or a single product that is a sunscreen and DEET combined. Using a DEET product along with a sunscreen may make the SPF less effective, and because sunscreen should be reapplied every 2 hours during the day (while DEET should not), a child may get overexposed to DEET with reapplication.

How Can I Baby-Proof My Garage?

As with indoor chemicals, **garage chemicals** such as lawn and garden fertilizers, herbicides, and pesticides can be dangerous if ingested. Locking them in cabinets and keeping them out of reach are the best ways to keep your kids safe.

Remember that toddlers often learn how to explore and find their way into the garage, so using baby-proofed doorknob covers to prevent entry is critically important.

To minimize another source of burns, children should be kept away **from outdoor fireplaces and grills** when they are in use and for several hours afterward when the grill or coals may still be hot.

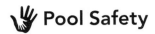 Pool Safety

What Are the Best Ways to Stay Safe Around Swimming Pools?

Swimming pools can provide another fun experience with your child, and a properly maintained chlorinated pool should be safe for most children. Many pediatricians don't recommend swimming pools for babies younger than 4 months, as they are less able to regulate their body temperature or hold their heads up well. In addition, the effects of chlorine exposure this young are not fully known, and new data suggest long chlorine exposure can be related to increased risk of bronchitis or similar respiratory conditions. All infants older than 4 months in swimming pools should have "touch supervision" at all times, which means an adult is never more than an arm's length away, even when the infant is using a life jacket or flotation device.

Private swimming pools at homes, as well as public facilities, should be secured with proper barriers, self-latching gates, and fencing to keep unsupervised children from entry. Even if doors leading to the pool are locked and have alarms, experts recommend to have the pool fenced in *separate* from the house and not include the house as one of the fence walls. Fences should be at least 4 feet high, have no more than 4 inches between the slats, and have no furniture pushed up against them that a child could climb up on to get over.

Should I Start Swimming Lessons for My Baby?

Some studies show a decreased risk for drowning in children as young as 1 year who received some formal swimming instruction (but no amount of instruction can completely eliminate the risk for drowning and should not be considered a way to "drown-proof" your child). Every child is different, and a parent is usually the best judge as to whether his child is ready for swim lessons. Swim lessons for babies younger than 1 year, however, have not shown any decreased risk for drowning.

Should We Circumcise Our Boy?

Circumcision is surgical removal of the foreskin surrounding the head of the penis and is a common surgical procedure performed on boys during the first few days of life. It is usually performed by a pediatrician or an obstetrician. Circumcision usually happens in the hospital on the last day of a newborn's stay there, and medicines such as lidocaine or a commercially available sugar solution given orally (during the procedure) and acetaminophen by mouth (after the procedure) are often given to minimize pain.

For parents, often the decision regarding whether to circumcise is made for social or religious reasons. In some religions, circumcision is expected. Socially, many parents opt to do whatever was done for family members. In the United States, circumcision is standard, but in some parts of the world, it is less commonly performed.

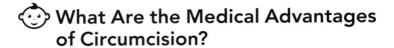 What Are the Medical Advantages of Circumcision?

The medical advantages of circumcision are believed to far outweigh the surgical risks. Studies have shown circumcised boys have a much lower risk for developing a urinary tract infection (UTI) in the first year of life (1 in 1,000 for circumcised infants versus 1 in 100 for non-circumcised). Later in life, circumcision is associated with a much lower risk for acquiring HIV and other sexually transmitted infections such as human papillomavirus, herpes, and syphilis.

How Do We Take Care of Circumcision After Surgery?

Care of the circumcision site is usually minimal. You should receive specific directions from your doctor, but generally experts recommend that petroleum jelly be applied to the tip of the penis with each diaper change for several days while it is healing. This will help keep the healing tip of the penis from sticking to the diaper. You should contact your pediatrician if you have any concerns after the procedure, including persistent bleeding, or if your baby is not urinating at least every 8 hours.

😊 Can We Circumcise Later?

For parents who choose not to circumcise, the option always exists to circumcise later. Really, it can be done at any time, but most parents who decide to proceed later do so when their boy is around 1 year old. For some medical conditions, delayed circumcision is preferred. One condition is hypospadias; the opening at the tip of the penis is on the underside of the head or shaft of the penis and is diagnosed by the pediatrician on examination. With hypospadias, circumcision is usually done when a baby is closer to 1 year. At this age, he is bigger, so the procedure can be done in a way that helps correct the hypospadias at the same time. Circumcision has a little more risk involved when done after the newborn period, but is still very safe, and is often done instead by a pediatric surgeon or pediatric urologist because it may require more anesthesia.

If you have questions or concerns, ask your doctor; either your obstetrician or pediatrician should be able to offer advice.

Is the Symptom My Baby Is Having Cause for Concern?

Why Is My Baby Sneezing?

Sneezing will happen every day for the first 1 or 2 months, especially the first week. Babies don't have seasonal or pet allergies this young, and infections usually come with other symptoms such as cough, fever, or fussiness. Dryness of the air we breathe can be irritating at first, so your newborn will likely make some mucus, and sneeze it up, to help lubricate her airways. Sneezing is also a built-in protective reflex: the nasal passages are so small in a newborn or young infant that even a small amount of mucus can cause congestion. Sneezing helps expel the mucus.

Do Hiccups Have Cures?

Hiccups are also common and have no proven cures despite all the advice you will receive. Some mothers may have even noticed that their baby had hiccups while in the womb. Unless the hiccups interfere with sleep or eating, medical attention is usually unnecessary.

Do I Need to Do Anything for My Baby's Peeling Skin?

Newborn skin often peels a few days after birth. If it gets red and irritated, try a little petroleum jelly. If not, just let it be. Don't over-wash; let those natural oils build up. A bath every 2 to 3 days is plenty.

What Can I Do for Baby Acne?

Acne usually shows up on the face after a few weeks and can last a few months. A gentle soap applied to a washcloth (or cotton square) and used on the face is fine. Medications are not needed; your baby's skin will adapt to its new environment, and acne resolves without scarring.

How Do I Know if My Baby's Poops Are Healthy?

Breastfed babies may not poop much the first couple days as their mothers' milk comes in. They may then poop 12 times a day for the next few weeks (bright yellow-mustard appearance) and may only poop once every few days by 3 to 4 months of age. This is all healthy. Formula-fed babies may poop 3 to 4 times a day, drop to once or twice a day, and hold steady every few days. As long as it's soft, and your baby is feeding well, wetting diapers, and not too fussy, all should be okay.

Is My Baby Constipated Because She Grunts and Strains When Pooping?

Many parents see their baby straining with bowel movements and worry about constipation. Usually the straining is not because the stools are hard but because their baby just isn't coordinated yet (we call this infantile dyschezia). Next time your baby is straining, try to bicycle those legs, and she should relax and pass the stools more easily.

Why Does He Have So Much Gas?

Most gas isn't swallowed but made internally by the partial digestion of formula or breast milk. Babies are just getting the hang of it. Don't worry at all the first 2 weeks. Gas isn't a problem; it's a sign that digestion is getting started. Gas typically peaks at 8 to 10 weeks of age and declines on its own. Don't start switching formulas every few days trying to find a remedy because your baby will take even longer to learn to digest his formula. You can try over-the-counter simethicone drops, but don't be surprised if your baby just needs to learn how to handle gas on his own. Swaddle and show love to him, and he'll get through this.

Is It Common for the Belly Button to Bleed or Ooze?

The umbilical cord stump typically separates or falls off around the second week of life but can do so as soon as a few days after birth or as late as a month after birth. During separation, seeing some yellow discharge and sometimes some bleeding is common, but this should stop easily and not continue. See your doctor if the healing stump continues to bleed or ooze, if the skin surrounding the umbilicus (belly button) becomes very red or warm, or if your baby has any fever.

What Should My Baby Be Doing as He or She Grows?

Some basic developmental milestones for each age are listed in this chapter. These lists are not requirements or assignments for children but, rather, a general picture of what most babies and toddlers are doing around these ages. Many children develop at their own pace, but because some delays can indicate developmental problems that can benefit from intervention (such as hearing loss or speech or swallowing problems), be sure to talk with your pediatrician if you think your child is not developing as she should be.

We will describe milestones by age based on the American Academy of Pediatrics and Bright Futures guidelines, which look at 4 basic categories of development: speech and communication skills, fine motor skills, gross motor skills, and social skills.

By 3 Months

Speech and communication.	Gurgling and cooing sounds.
Fine motor skills.	Opens hands and moves both arms and both legs equally.
Gross motor skills.	Holds head upright for a few seconds.
Social skills.	Begins to respond to your voice by making little noises (ie, squeaks, grunts, and coos) and making eye contact.

By 6 Months

Speech and communication.	Produces strings of cooing and vowel sounds.
Fine motor skills.	Plays with hands by touching them together and reaches for you.
Gross motor skills.	Tries to push upward with hands when on her stomach. Tries to bear weight on legs when held under her arms.
Social skills.	Turns head to sounds coming from a different room, reacts to emotions (eg, happiness, excitement, sadness) of others, relaxes when you read her a story, and notices herself in a mirror.

By 9 Months

Speech and communication.	Responds to quiet sounds and whispers with smiles and eye contact. Makes an attempt at saying words using vowels and consonants (eg, "mama," "dada," "baba," or "gaga").
Fine motor skills.	Tries to hold his bottle, drops or throws toys on purpose, and bangs and shakes his toys.
Gross motor skills.	Sits without support and without using his hands to hold himself up. Tries to crawl or creep on his hands and knees.
Social skills.	When shown a book, he gets excited and tries to grab and taste it. Often wary of people he doesn't know.

By 12 Months

Speech and communication.	Says at least one word other than "mama."
Fine motor skills.	Turns several pages when trying to turn pages in a book. Able to search for and find toys.
Gross motor skills.	Pulls up to standing position and walks holding onto furniture. Likes to explore objects and spaces.

| Social skills. | Likes to play peekaboo, turns her head in the direction of sound, and copies familiar behaviors, such as using a cup or telephone. Turns book faceup when upside down. |

By 18 Months

Speech and communication.	Says at least 4 to 10 words and can point to pictures you name in a book. Pretends to talk.
Fine motor skills.	Uses a cup without spilling and can take off his own shoes and feed himself.
Gross motor skills.	Walks across a large room without falling or wobbling from side to side.
Social skills.	Looks clearly to you in stressful situations and has temper tantrums.

By 24 Months

Speech and communication.	Says things such as "all gone," "go bye-bye," or other 2- to 3-word sentences and says about 50 words total. Tells you what she wants and repeats words others say.
Fine motor skills.	Takes off her own clothes (not just diapers, hats, and socks).
Gross motor skills.	Runs without falling often.
Social skills.	Looks at pictures in a book and pretends to read to you.

Are Immunizations Necessary (and Safe)?

Immunizations are such an important topic that squishing the high points into 1 or 2 pages is nearly impossible. But, in short, vaccines are one of the most powerful tools your pediatrician has to protect your child's life. In fact, many experts believe the 3 greatest achievements in halting the spread of disease are hand washing, pasteurization (sterilization of milk and other foods), and immunization.

💉 How Do Immunizations Work?

To simplify things a bit, your immune system has the ability to destroy germs that enter the body when you develop an infection. For example, when you catch a cold, your body is developing a "memory" of different aspects of the virus that caused the cold. Then, the next time your body catches the same virus, your immune system should remember it and destroy it before you experience symptoms. While catching an infection is one way to develop an immune response, some infections can be severe and potentially life threatening, and the benefit (future protection) is not worth the risk. That's where immunizations come in. They help educate your body into thinking it has caught a past infection. Immunizations are inactive versions or weakened strains of the germ. They do not cause the infection itself but do make your body develop a memory of an infection, so if you are ever infected with the real germ, your immune system is ready to attack.

Are Vaccines Safe?

Yes, vaccines are safe. You may have relatives or friends who fear vaccines and avoid them for their child. They may fear side effects of preservatives or the vaccines themselves, despite the prevailing scientific studies. Sadly, research has shown that delayed vaccines, or those not given at all, lead to unnecessary infections and deaths each year. Diseases that were nearly eradicated from the United States are now reoccurring because of some regional pockets of vaccine avoidance. Some parents believe that splitting vaccines which are usually given together will have some protective value; we now know it does not and creates unnecessary risks.

Do Vaccines Cause Autism?

No, vaccines do not cause autism. More than a decade ago, a widely-criticized article in a British medical journal described a potential link between vaccines and autism that led to vaccine avoidance. We now have years of studies, in countries across the globe, by universities and public health departments, all showing the same thing: vaccines have no relation to autism.

Vaccines are thoroughly studied, safety tested, and recommended by every major scientific body. Find a board-certified physician, and, most importantly, find a doctor you trust.

💉 How Do I Know What Vaccines My Child Needs?

Your pediatrician will help keep your child on an immunization schedule that will be coordinated with your checkups. The first vaccine, against the virus that causes hepatitis B, is usually given before a newborn leaves the hospital. Not every subsequent checkup comes with vaccines, but at the beginning, it will seem like it. Most vaccines come as shots; some are oral (the rotavirus vaccine for babies) and some are nasal (the flu vaccine for many children older than 2 years). Some vaccines are given on the same day, and some are even multiple vaccines combined into the same shot, such as the MMR vaccine, which stands for measles, mumps, and rubella. We know this sounds like a lot, but rest assured, vaccines that are given together are safety tested in combination for this very reason. Although the amount of vaccines may seem like a heavy load for a baby's immune system, in fact, a baby often is exposed to many more germs or dietary proteins each day than in all of her vaccines.

Here are a few tips to help prepare for immunization.

- **Immunization schedule.** Trust the American Academy of Pediatrics immunization schedule and your doctor. The schedule is created to help your baby be as protected as possible, without major side effects, and your doctor will know if significant side effects are developing in her patients.
- **Acetaminophen.** Discuss with your doctor if you can give acetaminophen to your baby after the shots (or ibuprofen if your baby is older than 6 months), but don't give it before you come. You don't want to mask a fever when the nurse checks for one.
- **Records.** Ask for a copy of your baby's shot record each visit. You may not think you need it, but it's much easier to get it that day than to come back later (and some doctor's offices charge a small fee to get shot records if it's not part of your visit).

Is My Baby Sleeping Enough? When Will We Sleep Longer?

Sleep is one of the greatest areas of concern for new families and is an important part of a baby's life. Each age group comes with its own common challenges, so let's see if we can shed some light on these questions.

🧸 First 2 Weeks

How Much Sleep Is Common?

New parents are often concerned about how much their new baby sleeps when he comes home from the hospital. Some will sleep 19, 20, or even 22 hours a day and only wake up to feed. This is common and okay. Newborns have been used to sleeping in a dark, quiet womb and were getting continuous feedings through their umbilical cord. So, day and night, as well as feeding cycles, are new adjustments for them. As long as the feedings are going well and your baby is not too fussy, you are in good shape.

🐻 At 2 Weeks to 2 Months

Why Does My Baby Wake Up So Often?

Babies 2 weeks to 2 months old are just learning how to soothe themselves, need to eat frequently, and will surprise you with how often they poop. Feed your baby when he's hungry, change him when needed, and let him sleep whenever he'd like in his bassinet or crib, with no blankets or stuffed animals around to risk suffocation. Two big tips for this age are to establish a nighttime routine (such as a bath, cuddling time, and consistent times for falling asleep) and to learn how to soothe your baby with swaddling and rocking.

🐻 At 2 to 6 Months

Do I Spoil Her if I Pick Her Up When She Cries While Trying to Sleep?

No. Babies 2 to 6 months are learning to self-soothe, so you've got a range of options when it comes to sleep. Some people continue with their unstructured sleep, as described, but many start thinking about sleep-training methods, which include everything on the spectrum, from the cry-it-out method on one end to attachment parenting on the other.

Cry-It-Out Method

Proponents of this method have demonstrated effectiveness of letting a baby fuss on her own for slowly increasing periods (eg,

1 minute for a few nights, 2 minutes for a few nights) in hopes that she learns to soothe herself in her crib.

Attachment Parenting

Supporters of attachment parenting feel you violate your baby's trust if you let her cry without being right there to help and if you don't offer ideas to help her learn some self-soothing skills without crying.

Many parents end up falling somewhere between these positions, and, in the end, studies suggest that consistency is key. Total sleep may decline to 12 to 15 hours per day during this phase. Find a method that works for you, and stick to it! Also, naps start to become more predictable during this time, usually settling at 2 to 3 naps per day, each lasting 1 to 2 hours. Follow your baby's schedule during the day, and play with her after she eats before laying her down for her nap.

🐻 At 6 to 12 Months

What Do I Need to Do to Help Him Learn to Sleep?

If you haven't thought about sleep training yet, and are hoping to do so, 6 to 12 months is the ideal time. As your baby's needs change, you'll see a lot more curiosity and will likely see more nighttime awakenings, and you want nights to be a well-settled event at this point. Don't be surprised if new changes in development, such as in feeding pattern, mobility, and teething, all come with short periods of worsened nighttime sleep. Stick to your plan. Comfort briefly while your baby is in his crib, and emphasize routine for your sake and for your baby's. Healthy sleep involves periods of waking briefly, and falling back to sleep, so those little noises, whimpers, or movements on the monitor are to be expected; babies don't lie still all night. In fact, those in this age group often sleep in the 12 to 14 hours per day range, wake several times per night (and, hopefully, fall right back asleep), and often drop down to 1 or 2 naps per day.

🐻 At 12 to 24 Months

How Do I Help My Child Stay Asleep and Return to Sleep?

Most of the time after the first birthday, sleep is less of a concern, but new issues may arise from time to time. Here is a list of some of the more common questions we receive and how we address them with parents.

Why Does My Baby Wake Up Crying at Night?

If your baby is not hungry, wet, or soiled, you may be hearing the cries of night terrors (not nightmares). These sound similar and sometimes are hard to tell apart. Nightmares usually happen later in the night when the child is dreaming, while a night terror often happens earlier in the night when the child is in deep sleep but not dreaming. The biggest difference for your child is with a nightmare, children will usually wake up scared and not want to go back to sleep, which will likely occur when they are older than 2 years. With a night terror (which can occur before 2), they may be screaming or seem scared when they are asleep, but once they wake up, they will have no memory of it and will not be scared anymore. In fact, a night terror is usually more frightening for the parent than the child, and the child will go back to sleep easily. Either way, as a parent, your instinct will probably be to go in and check on your child. With a night terror, children will go back to sleep on their own and will not need much comforting from you. With a nightmare, however, reassure them, help them realize whatever they were scared of was not real, and give them some comfort by eliminating anything they are scared of (eg, shadows, open closet doors). Also, letting a babysitter know about these if your child has them frequently is a good idea.

My Toddler Does Not Want to Go to Sleep! Is This Common?

You may have conquered the bedtime routine during the first year, but expect other bumps in the road. At times your child will get out of the usual routine, and you may find it necessary to retrain her sleep habits. Your child now may have a little more willpower than before and may be more aware of other distractions in the house.

How Do I Establish a Bedtime Routine?

Each night, to establish a bedtime routine, give your child a bath, read her favorite book, and sing the same bedtime song. Be sure to keep the activities the same way at the same time every night. These cues will help trigger a reminder that it really is bedtime. Also, set the bedroom up with the same favorite items, such as a favorite blanket, stuffed animal, or night-light, or other cues that are associated with bedtime.

Is Having Playtime Right Before Bedtime Okay?

Avoid too much roughhousing and physical playtime right before bedtime, which may get your child worked up. The bedtime routine should be as minimally stimulating as possible. Also, avoid electronics; even though you may have a movie or game on the tablet that your child enjoys, studies show screen time is actually stimulating and makes going to sleep harder.

My Child Has Been Fussy All Night. Can He Sleep in My Bed?

For the best-quality sleep for everyone in the family, try to resist letting your child sleep in your bed. Even though that may seem like the easiest option at 1:00 am, or if he is extremely fussy, letting it persist will just result in poor sleep for both you and him and may lead to difficulty sleeping in his crib or bassinet.

What Is SIDS?

☪ What Is SIDS?

Sudden infant death syndrome (SIDS) is a rare condition that results in the unexpected death of an infant younger than 1 year. It usually happens before 6 months, and the peak of occurrence is between 2 to 4 months.

☪ What Causes SIDS? Can I Prevent It?

While the cause of SIDS has no single explanation, experts have theories as to why SIDS happens and have determined well-known risk factors. Some of the risk factors are generally unavoidable, including prematurity, low birth weight, poverty, and race. Other risk factors, however, can be controlled to reduce the risk of SIDS.

- **Don't smoke in the home.** Infants who are around cigarette smoke, not only active (visible) smoke but also passive (the presence of smoke on clothing and bedding), have a much higher risk of SIDS. We recommend no smoking around newborns or infants, and avoid spending time with other caregivers who smoke.

- **Put your baby in the proper sleeping position.** All infants should sleep on their back. This debate often causes stress with grandparents who remember the days when new parents were told to place infants on their belly to sleep because of the presumed risk of aspiration from vomiting. However, there has been a 40% decrease in SIDS over the past 20 years since the Safe to Sleep campaign (an expansion of the Back to Sleep campaign).

- **Avoid co-sleeping.** Having your infant cuddled up in bed with you may feel comforting and protective. Sometimes keeping him in bed if he falls asleep while feeding just seems easier. Unfortunately, co-sleeping is becoming the most frequently found risk factor contributing to SIDS. We encourage parents to let their infant sleep as close to them as they want but in a separate bassinet or crib and not in bed with them. Infants should not sleep on a sofa, chair, or any other location not designed for infant sleep.

Part 3

Pediatric Checkups

Introduction

Understanding Growth Charts

What Is a Growth Chart?

At every checkup, your pediatrician will plot your baby's growth statistics (curves) on something called a growth chart. This chart is one of your doctor's most important tools and can help identify problems with health and nutrition. Figures 3-1 and 3-2 are examples of current growth charts for boys and for girls respectively under the age of 2.

How Does It Work?

When your pediatrician shows you your baby's growth chart, you will see a series of curves—height, weight, and head circumference for an infant and height, weight, and body mass index for a child. Also, charts are separated based on sex (and even special populations, such as premature infants). The curves will have a central darkest line to represent the 50th percentile—the average, or most common, reading. Other parallel curves will be above and below the 50th percentile line to represent other percentiles, from 2nd up to 98th. When plotting growth curves on the chart, the values for that day are only partially helpful; what your pediatrician will track is how your child's percentiles change from visit to visit over time. Every child is different; that's why such a large zone is considered typical. Ideally, your infant's or child's curves should plot within this zone and, over time, her growth percentiles should mirror the center line. Your pediatrician may become concerned if

- Your child's percentiles cross over 2 of the percentile lines or fall above or below the typical ranges for the curve. Such rapid changes could indicate a medical condition or dietary issues leading to unhealthy growth.
- Your child's percentiles are tracking in different directions (eg, the weight percentile is going up, but the height percentile is going down). This may also indicate a medical condition unrelated to diet.

The most common reasons a child's growth percentiles will show unusual change are inaccurate measurement and inaccurate plotting. Now that many doctors use electronic medical records, plotting not only is more accurate (assuming no mechanical error) but will also be calculated based on exactly how old your infant is (eg, 6 months and 3 weeks). With paper plotting, age tends to be rounded off to the nearest month (if your doctor thinks this is the 6-month checkup, he may round back to 6 months even if your infant is 7 or 8 months).

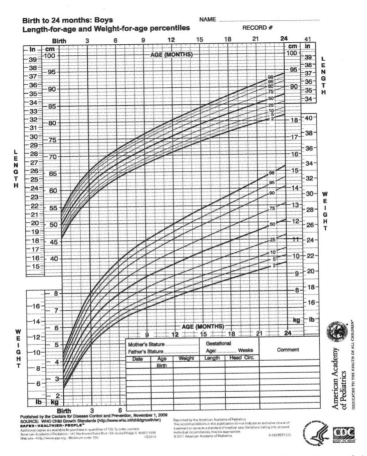

Figure 3-1 Sample growth chart for weight and length for boys (birth to 24 months).

Developed by the National Center for Health Statistics in collaboration with the National Center for Chronic Disease Prevention and Health Promotion (2000). http://www.cdc.gov/growthcharts

Reprinted by the American Academy of Pediatrics

The recommendations in this publication do not indicate an exclusive course of treatment or serve as a standard of medical care. Variations, taking into account individual circumstances, may be appropriate.

© American Academy of Pediatrics

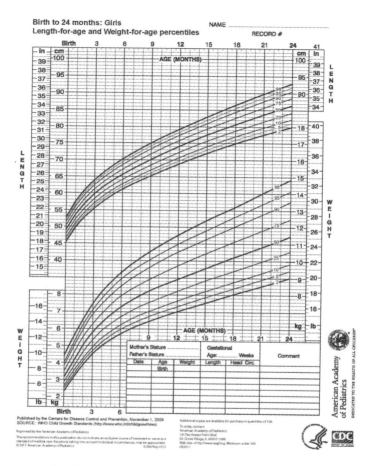

Figure 3.2 Sample growth chart for weight and length for girls (birth to 24 months).

Developed by the National Center for Health Statistics in collaboration with the National Center for Chronic Disease Prevention and Health Promotion (2000). http://www.cdc.gov/growthcharts

Reprinted by the American Academy of Pediatrics

The recommendations in this publication do not indicate an exclusive course of treatment or serve as a standard of medical care. Variations, taking into account individual circumstances, may be appropriate.

© American Academy of Pediatrics

About Pediatric Checkups

Pediatric checkups are a time for your doctor to evaluate growth, development, and overall health of your baby. You may be given some questionnaires to fill out to address your baby's development or risks of medical issues (eg, lead exposure, tuberculosis exposure). Your baby should get a full examination by your doctor with each of these checkups. Pediatricians follow a standardized schedule to keep a close tab on your baby's growth and development. Many of the checkups coincide with getting vaccines or laboratory work; some do not.

Each checkup is a time for your doctor to review your child's growth chart and see if anything that has happened since your child's last checkup warrants further review. In between checkups, your child may have seen your regular pediatrician, his partners, or staff at an urgent care setting for an ear infection or other illness. You may have been to a subspecialist, who sent your doctor a note he wants to review with you, or your child may be on medications that should be reviewed for dosing changes or to be stopped.

At a checkup is the best time for you to bring up any questions you have about how to care for your baby. This may include areas of concerns at home (eg, feeding, sleep) or concerns regarding aspects of medical care (eg, vaccines, referrals to subspecialists). You may also have questions that you didn't think warranted a separate visit or phone call. Writing these down is a good idea, as you may forget to ask when the appointment comes around. Also, don't feel embarrassed that your question is too silly or unimportant; a parent's intuition has real merit. Your concern may indeed turn out to be about something completely normal.

Like the rest of the book, we'll cover the checkups through 2 years of age, which will detail each visit, from preparation, to during, to after. Also, each checkup chapter is followed by a health record section, where you can record your child's percentiles, questions and answers from the visit, and plans for the next few weeks or months.

Keeping these appointments is important, even if vaccines aren't scheduled to happen and you think your child is developing well. Your doctor is trained to look for certain developmental milestones or health problems at each checkup (both on history and examination) that you may have not anticipated. If you have opinions or thoughts about your child's progress, if you need any referral, or if you need paperwork filled out for day care, checkups are the best time to get them addressed.

Here's a quick overview of the checkup timeline.

- First checkup (usually 1 to 3 days after leaving the hospital)
- 2 to 4 weeks
- 2 months
- 4 months

- 6 months
- 9 months
- 12 months
- 15 months
- 18 months
- 2 years
- 2½ years
- 3 years
- 4 years

Don't forget to take pictures before each visit! You'll enjoy looking back and seeing your bundle of joy grow over the next two years.

The First-Week Checkup

Before the Visit

You are home from the hospital with your new bundle of joy and may have a few questions. Write them down in this book, and bring it with you; these questions will help organize the visit and allow you to get answers to your primary concerns. The hospital staff will tell you when you need to follow up with your pediatrician and will generally give you the office phone number or make the appointment for you. Give yourself plenty of time (many people suggest an hour) to get ready with diapers, car seats, directions, breastfeeding covers or bottles, and required paperwork.

Questions for Today's Checkup

1.

2.

3.

👨‍⚕️ Bring With You

- A list of any medications or problems you may have had during your pregnancy or delivery
- Any paperwork you may have picked up from the office before delivery (If you can complete it at home, you will save yourself time in the waiting room.)
- Any paperwork that the hospital staff gave you at discharge

👨‍⚕️ During the Visit

➡ If you have not met your pediatrician before this visit, you will get your first chance to see the office, the staff, and him. The staff will likely ask you basic questions about your pregnancy and your baby's delivery. Then they will ask you to undress your baby for weight, length, and head measurements and to take a rectal temperature. These steps will help ensure consistent accurate measurements, which are entered onto the growth chart to start tracking your baby's growth. It is not unusual for a baby to have lost weight during this time and to have jaundice (be yellow in color).

➡ Your doctor should perform a full examination of your baby, including looking for evidence of jaundice, dehydration, heart or lung problems, or any birthmarks. Many newborns require jaundice measurements from a heel sample at this visit.

➡ Feel free to ask your doctor any question, and show him your list of questions early, as it will help guide your discussion. Take notes on what your pediatrician advises. You may want to revisit those answers later.

➡ Your doctor should advise you on some baby basics— healthy feeding, elimination and sleep, safety, starting vitamin D, umbilical and circumcision care (if needed), ways to avoid illnesses, and ways to reach the office with any questions.

After the Visit

☐ If you need help finding a lactation consultant, ask who your doctor recommends.

☐ Set up your 2- to 4-week follow-up visit (or any other recommended visit) now while appointments are available.

☐ Anticipate a call with the jaundice test result, and if the level is elevated, your newborn may need photo (light) therapy or a recheck the following morning. The office will help set these up.

☐ Start reading to your baby to help with her language skills and brain development.

Baby Health Record: First-Week Checkup

Baby's Name:

Date:
Office:
Pediatrician Name:

Birth Weight:
Hospital Discharge Weight:
Today's Weight:
Bilirubin Level:
Did this require any therapy or changes to baby's feeding patterns?

Feeding Habits:

Elimination Habits:

Sleep Habits:

Questions We Addressed:

1.

2.

3.

Things to Do After This Visit:

1.

2.

3.

Notes:

The 2- to 4-Week Checkup

Your new baby will be changing every day, and, as he develops, your comfort level and questions will change as well.

Before the Visit

Observe any feeding patterns, sleeping patterns, changes in bowel movements, and wet diapers, and write down any question you have in the space provided.

Questions for Today's Checkup

1.

2.

3.

Bring With You

■ Your list of questions

■ Any medications or supplements you or your baby may be taking (such as the vitamin D drops recommended for breastfeeding infants)

During the Visit

➡ Your infant's temperature will be taken, and his weight, length, and head will be measured and plotted on the growth chart, as they were at the first visit.

➡ Your discussion with your infant's doctor will likely center around your baby's growth and development, with a focus on concerns at this young age that could indicate a problem with nutrition and feeding. Safety, sleep, and elimination will be key topics, as well as any topics you bring with you.

➡ Your infant may be due for a hepatitis B vaccine, although the recommended timing of this vaccine is flexible at this age if the first dose was given in the hospital at birth.

➡ Ask your doctor about the newborn metabolic screening, as results should now be available.

After the Visit

☐ Schedule your follow-up appointment (which will usually be at 2 months of age).

☐ Read What Should I Know About Breastfeeding or Formula Feeding? on page 35 and What Should My Baby Be Doing as He or She Grows? on page 64 about infant development.

☐ Note any concerns you have about your baby as she grows.

☐ If you're breastfeeding your baby, remember to take your prenatal vitamins and give a vitamin D supplement (only if breastfeeding) directly to your baby.

Baby Health Record:
2- to 4-Week Checkup

Baby's Name:

Date:

Office:

Pediatrician Name:

Today's Weight: _____, which is the _____ percentile.

Today's Length: _____, which is the _____ percentile.

Today's Head Size: _____, which is the _____ percentile.

Feeding Habits:

Elimination Habits:

Sleep Habits:

Milestones Noted So Far:

Questions We Addressed:

1.

2.

3.

Things to Do After This Visit:

1.

2.

3.

Notes:

The 2-Month Checkup

Many 2-month-olds are either breastfeeding 8 or more times per day or bottle-feeding 6 to 8 times per day. Many wet diapers are to be expected, and bowel movement frequency can range from several per day to one every several days. Many parents start to notice routines taking shape at home, and if you have questions about helping your baby settle into that routine, bring those to today's visit.

Before the Visit

Every baby develops at her own pace. Take note of any questions you have about development.

Questions for Today's Checkup

1.

2.

3.

Bring With You

- Extra diapers and wipes, as well as acetaminophen for use after today's vaccines.
- Your list of questions and notes about your baby's development, feeding, elimination, and sleeping patterns
- A cover to breastfeed your baby soon after the visit, or a bottle to give, to help distract and soothe her
- Forms required by child care facilities, if needed

During the Visit

➡ Expect a full set of measurements (ie, temperature, height, weight, and head circumference), as in the first few visits. Your pediatrician should discuss your concerns, review safety and baby care, and fully examine your baby. Now is a good chance to mention any plans to return to work and discuss your options about child care.

➡ For this visit, the Centers for Disease Control and Prevention and the American Academy of Pediatrics recommend immunization against polio, diphtheria, tetanus, pertussis, pneumococcal disease, *Haemophilus influenzae* type b disease, rotavirus disease, and hepatitis B. Several of these can be given in combination to minimize the number of vaccines given at one time.

➡ Do not give acetaminophen in advance, which suppresses fever. Your doctor will want to know if your baby has a fever at the checkup and may even delay vaccines if it is high.

➡ Screening questionnaires may be given to focus on exposure to lead (a toxic metal in old paint and a few other sources) or tuberculosis (a lung infection).

After the Visit

☐ Give acetaminophen, dosed according to your baby's weight, up to every 4 to 6 hours if she has a fever or is crying more than usual after vaccinations. If she's happy, she doesn't need any specific treatment.

☐ Schedule the 4-month appointment, if possible.

☐ Continue your nutrition as before, and continue your vitamin D drops if you are breastfeeding your baby.

☐ Start anticipating your baby's increasing strength; she may try to start rolling and needs to be closely watched while being changed or bathed.

☐ Continue reading to your baby, even though she just hears your voice.

Baby Health Record: 2-Month Checkup

Baby's Name:

Date:

Office:

Pediatrician Name:

Today's Weight: _____, which is the _____ percentile.

Today's Length: _____, which is the _____ percentile.

Today's Head Size: _____, which is the _____ percentile.

Feeding Habits:

Elimination Habits:

Sleep Habits:

Milestones Noted So Far:

Questions We Addressed:

1.

2.

3.

Things to Do After This Visit:

1.

2.

3.

Notes:

The 4-Month Checkup

Four months of age is often called the beginning of the Golden Age of Infancy, as babies have generally figured out how to best digest breast milk or formula, are getting stronger, and are smiling more. As they improve their ability to reach and hold, as well as roll their bodies and push up when lying down, their curiosity grows, and they can start to soothe themselves when fussy. This is a great age to read and sing to your baby, as she learns to explore and experience her world.

Before the Visit

Review What Should My Baby Be Doing as He or She Grows? on page 64 about developmental milestones to get a sense of how most 4-month-olds are developing.

Questions for Today's Checkup

1.

2.

3.

👨‍⚕️ Bring With You

- Extra diapers and wipes, as well as acetaminophen for use after today's vaccines
- Your list of questions about your baby's developmental, feeding, elimination, and sleeping patterns
- A cover to breastfeed your baby soon after the visit, or a bottle to give, to help distract and soothe her
- Books for the waiting room
- Forms required by child care facilities, if needed

👨‍⚕️ During the Visit

➡ Expect a full set of measurements (ie, temperature, height, weight, and head circumference), as in the first few visits. Your doctor should discuss with you concerns on your list, review safety and baby care, and fully examine your baby. This is a good chance to mention any plans to return to work and discuss any concerns about child care options. If you already returned to work, talk about your experience, transition, and any possible concerns.

➡ Be sure to discuss upcoming feeding plans. The American Academy of Pediatrics and World Health Organization recommend exclusively breastfeeding until your baby is 6 months of age, but if you have questions about starting solid foods earlier, discuss these with your pediatrician.

➡ For this visit, the Centers for Disease Control and Prevention and the American Academy of Pediatrics recommend immunization for polio, diphtheria, tetanus, pertussis, pneumococcal disease, *Haemophilus influenzae* type b disease, and rotavirus disease, as well as any vaccines that were not able to be given at a previous checkup. Several of these can be given in combination to minimize the number of immunizations.

➡ Don't give acetaminophen in advance, which suppresses fever. Your doctor will want to know if your baby has a fever at the checkup and may even delay vaccines if it is high.

➡ Screening questionnaires may be given to focus on exposure to lead (a toxic metal in old paint and a few other sources) or tuberculosis (a lung infection).

After the Visit

☐ Schedule your infant's 6-month visit before leaving the office.

☐ Give acetaminophen, dosed according to your infant's weight, up to every 4 to 6 hours if she has a fever or is in pain after immunizations. If she's happy, she doesn't need any medication.

☐ Continue your nutrition as before, and continue your vitamin D drops if you are breastfeeding your baby.

☐ Read to your baby every day!

Baby Health Record: 4-Month Checkup

Baby's Name:

Date:
Office:
Pediatrician Name:

Today's Weight: _____, which is the _____ percentile.
Today's Length: _____, which is the _____ percentile.
Today's Head Size: _____, which is the _____ percentile.

Feeding Habits:

Elimination Habits:

Sleep Habits:

Milestones Noted So Far:

Questions We Addressed:

1.

2.

3.

Things to Do After This Visit:

1.

2.

3.

Notes:

The 6-Month Checkup

At 6 months of age, babies are generally starting to sit up (at first supported by you or in a high chair, then on their own), show their personalities, and show interest in what you're saying and eating. As an infant learns to look and observe, he wants to be stimulated and engaged, so your focus as a parent will turn to helping him stay safe during his new experiences.

Before the Visit

Babies often are introduced to solid foods between 4 to 6 months. Read Baby Foods: When and How Do We Start Solid Foods? on page 43, and note any questions about how you plan to feed your baby.

Questions for Today's Checkup

1.

2.

3.

Bring With You

- Diapers and wipes, as well as acetaminophen or ibuprofen (now that your infant is 6 months of age) for use after today's immunizations, if needed
- Your list of questions about your baby's developmental, feeding, elimination, and sleeping patterns
- A cover to breastfeed your baby soon after the visit, or a bottle to give, to help distract and soothe him
- Toys or books to entertain your baby in the waiting or examination room
- Forms required by child care facilities, if needed

During the Visit

➡ Your discussion today will focus largely on feeding complementary solid foods and thinking about sleep patterns for infants.

➡ Expect a full set of measurements (ie, temperature, height, weight, and head circumference), as in the first few visits. Your pediatrician should discuss with you concerns on your list, review safety and baby care, and fully examine your baby.

➡ Baby's developmental milestones become more obvious (eg, sitting with support, making noises), so your pediatrician should evaluate your baby's development to be sure it is progressing as it should and to give advice or assistance if not.

➡ The Centers for Disease Control and Prevention and the American Academy of Pediatrics recommend immunization for polio, diphtheria, tetanus, pertussis, pneumococcal disease, *Haemophilus influenzae* type b disease, and rotavirus disease, as well as any vaccines that were not able to be given at a previous checkup.

➡ If flu vaccine season is underway (usually September through April), the Centers for Disease Control and Prevention and the American Academy of Pediatrics also recommend an infant dose of flu vaccine, with a repeat infant dose at least 1 month later. This second visit is not usually another well-child visit but, rather, a brief visit for the vaccine only.

➡ Don't give acetaminophen in advance, which suppresses fever. Your doctor will want to know if your baby has a fever at the checkup and may even delay vaccines if it is high.

➡ Screening questionnaires may be given to focus on your baby's exposure to lead (a toxic metal in old paint and a few other sources) or tuberculosis (a lung infection).

After the Visit

☐ Schedule your baby's 9-month visit and follow-up flu vaccine in 1 month, if needed.

☐ Give acetaminophen or ibuprofen, dosed according to your baby's weight, up to every 4 to 6 hours if he has a fever or appears to be in pain (fussy or crying) after immunizations.

☐ If you are breastfeeding your infant, continue your prenatal vitamins and continue to give your baby a multivitamin supplement to help provide enough zinc, iron, and vitamin D for your baby. Formula-fed infants do not need supplemental vitamins, as these are included in the formula.

☐ Read to your baby every day!

☐ Set a goal of indoor and outdoor baby-proofing and safety before your baby is 9 months and mobile. If it's summertime, read How Do I Keep My Baby Safe Outside? on page 52 about outdoor safety.

Baby Health Record: 6-Month Checkup

Baby's Name:

Date:
Office:
Pediatrician Name:

Today's Weight: _____, which is the _____ percentile.
Today's Length: _____, which is the _____ percentile.
Today's Head Size: _____, which is the _____ percentile.

Feeding Habits:

Elimination Habits:

Sleep Habits:

Milestones Noted So Far:

Questions We Addressed:

1.

2.

3.

Things to Do After This Visit:

1.

2.

3.

Notes:

The 9-Month Checkup

Nine months of age marks the beginning of mobility (ie, crawling, cruising, and, eventually, walking) for some babies, and the focus of parenthood shifts to safety for many parents.

Before the Visit

Note any concerns you have about your baby's development, and write down any additional questions about your baby's feeding, sleeping, or elimination patterns, as well as any notes on safety concerns.

Questions for Today's Checkup

1.

2.

3.

👶 Bring With You

- Diapers and wipes and a cover to breastfeed your baby, or a bottle to give, soon after the visit, if immunizations were needed
- Your list of questions and notes about your baby's developmental, feeding, elimination, and sleeping patterns, as well as safety concerns
- A few toys and books for the waiting and examination room
- Forms required by child care facilities, if needed

👶 During the Visit

➡ Your discussion today will focus on your questions, on the change in your baby's nutrition, and on the need to provide the safest possible environment for your baby.

➡ Expect a full set of measurements (ie, temperature, height, weight, and head circumference), as in the first few visits. Your doctor should discuss with you concerns on your list, review safety and baby care, and fully examine your baby.

➡ As at the 6-month checkup, milestones and development will be assessed to ensure that no further therapies or assistance need to be provided at this stage.

➡ Screening questionnaires may again be given to focus on exposure to lead or tuberculosis. Per American Academy of Pediatrics guidelines, developmental screening should be done at 9, 18, and 30 months of age.

➡ Ask your pediatrician for his advice on starting sippy cups and appropriate finger foods to encourage infants to take a larger role in their own feedings.

➡ If it is flu vaccine season (and was not at the last checkup), the Centers for Disease Control and Prevention and the American Academy of Pediatrics recommend the flu vaccine (in season, with a repeat infant vaccine in 1 month) but no other vaccines unless your baby needs to catch up on ones missed at an earlier visit.

➡ As always, do not give acetaminophen in advance, which suppresses fever. Your doctor will want to know if your baby has a fever at the checkup and may even delay vaccines if it is high.

👨‍⚕️ After the Visit

☐ Schedule your 12-month checkup and follow-up flu vaccine, if needed

☐ Recognize new skills as new opportunities to teach and engage your infant, and be aware that his increasing mobility will require efforts to keep him safe indoors and out.

☐ Read to your baby every day, and avoid exposing your baby to television or computer screen time. These few steps can set the stage for better development and learning for the future.

☐ Your baby may be ready to start to eat 3 meals of thicker and chunkier (stage 3) baby foods per day, with snacks between meals, and will likely be drinking less breast milk or formula at this age, as solid foods play a larger role in his nutrition.

☐ Review How Do I Baby-Proof My Home? on page 48 and How Do I Keep My Baby Safe Outside? on page 52 for indoor and outdoor safety.

Baby Health Record: 9-Month Checkup

Baby's Name:

Date:
Office:
Pediatrician Name:

Today's Weight: _____, which is the _____ percentile.
Today's Length: _____, which is the _____ percentile.
Today's Head Size: _____, which is the _____ percentile.

Feeding Habits:

Elimination Habits:

Sleep Habits:

Milestones Noted So Far:

Questions We Addressed:

1.

2.

3.

Things to Do After This Visit:

1.

2.

3.

Notes:

The 12-Month Checkup

Your baby is 12 months old! Now it's really game on; the house has to be baby-proofed, and the habits and expectations you set will make the rest of toddlerhood easier. Consistent sleep habits, reading time, and avoidance of television and other digital media are critically important steps to assist in your baby's development.

Before the Visit

Check What Should My Baby Be Doing as He or She Grows? on page 64 for developmental milestones at this age, note any concerns you have about your baby's development, and write down any additional questions you may have.

Questions for Today's Checkup

1.

2.

3.

👨‍⚕️ Bring With You

- Diapers and wipes, as well as acetaminophen or ibuprofen (now that your infant is older than 6 months)
- Your list of questions or concerns
- Toys and books for any needed waits

👨‍⚕️ During the Visit

➡ Your discussion today will continue to focus on nutrition, development, and safety and will likely review some typical milestones for this age.

➡ Expect a full set of measurements (ie, temperature, height, weight, and head circumference), as in the first few visits. Your doctor should discuss with you concerns on your list, review safety and baby care, and fully examine your baby.

➡ Your baby may have blood tests for lead or hemoglobin.

➡ Ask your pediatrician if she recommends a daily vitamin.

➡ Ask your pediatrician for advice on transitioning to table foods, toddler cups, and whole cow's milk.

➡ At this visit, there can be some variation in the immunization schedule, depending on your pediatrician and which vaccines she uses. In addition to the pneumococcal immunization, doctors may start the measles-mumps-rubella and varicella immunizations and may complete the *Haemophilus influenzae* type B vaccine series and start the hepatitis A vaccine series.

→ If it is flu vaccine season (and was not at the last checkup), the Centers for Disease Control and Prevention and the American Academy of Pediatrics recommend an infant dose of flu vaccine, with a single repeat infant dose at least 1 month later.

→ Don't give acetaminophen in advance, which suppresses fever. Your doctor will want to know if your infant has a fever at the checkup and may even delay vaccines if your baby's temperature is elevated.

After the Visit

☐ Schedule your 15-month visit and follow-up flu vaccine, if needed.

☐ If needed, you may give acetaminophen or ibuprofen, dosed according to your baby's weight, up to every 4 to 6 hours if she has a fever or is in pain after immunizations.

☐ Find a way to incorporate your baby's new skills and coordination in your play. Offer new toys that use her increased dexterity, and read from books with bright colors and new textures to stimulate your baby.

☐ Your baby will be transitioning to table foods and whole cow's milk unless feeding problems or food allergies are encountered.

Baby Health Record: 12-Month Checkup

Baby's Name:

Date:
Office:
Pediatrician Name:

Today's Weight: _____, which is the _____ percentile.
Today's Length: _____, which is the _____ percentile.
Today's Head Size: _____, which is the _____ percentile.

Feeding Habits:

Elimination Habits:

Sleep Habits:

Milestones Noted So Far:

Questions We Addressed:

1.

2.

3.

Things to Do After This Visit:

1.

2.

3.

Notes:

The 15-Month Checkup

Toddlers at 15 months old start to know what they want to do and not do, and some signs of independence become obvious. Communication skills may increase, including gesturing and babbling, and will improve the more you engage and talk to your toddler. Your focus will be on maintaining a safe environment and deciding on boundaries that give you peace of mind and also give your child some choices with what to play with and do during the day.

Before the Visit

Check What Should My Baby Be Doing as He or She Grows? on page 64 for developmental milestones. Keep track of how much whole cow's milk and food your child has eaten and how much your child is sleeping so you can discuss these.

Questions for Today's Checkup

1.

2.

3.

🧑‍⚕️ Bring With You

- Your list of questions
- Snacks and milk in case you want to soothe your child after immunizations
- Books or toys for in the waiting or examination room (One-year-olds need more distraction than anyone.)
- Forms required by child care facilities, if needed
- Diapers and wipes, as well as acetaminophen or ibuprofen

🧑‍⚕️ During the Visit

➡ Your discussion today will continue to focus on safety and nutrition and start to focus more on communication milestones, which are important signs that your toddler is thriving.

➡ Expect a full set of measurements (ie, temperature, height, weight, and head circumference), as in the first few visits. Your doctor should discuss with you concerns on your list, review safety and toddler care, and fully examine your toddler.

➡ At this visit, there may be variation in the immunization schedule, and your toddler will likely complete the diphtheria-tetanus-pertussis vaccine series, as well as vaccines that were not able to be received at the 12-month checkup.

➡ If it is flu vaccine season (and it was not at the last checkup), the Centers of Disease Control and Prevention and the American Academy of Pediatrics also recommend an infant dose of flu vaccine, with a repeat infant dose at least 1 month later.

➡ Don't give acetaminophen or ibuprofen in advance, which suppresses fever. Your doctor will want to know if your toddler has a fever at the checkup and may even delay vaccines if it is high.

👪 After the Visit

☐ Schedule your 18-month visit and follow-up flu vaccine if needed.

☐ Observe your child's developing coordination and mobility, and look for obvious improvements.

☐ Continue to focus on nutrition, with table foods and whole cow's milk being the likely dominant part of your child's healthy eating. Your pediatrician may give you strategies to transition to these table foods.

Toddler Health Record: 15-Month Checkup

Toddler's Name:

Date:
Office:
Pediatrician Name:

Today's Weight: _____, which is the _____ percentile.
Today's Length: _____, which is the _____ percentile.
Today's Head Size: _____, which is the _____ percentile.

Feeding Habits:

Elimination Habits:

Sleep Habits:

Milestones Noted So Far:

Questions We Addressed:

1.

2.

3.

Things to Do After This Visit:

1.

2.

3.

Notes:

The 18-Month Checkup

Many toddlers are developing independence as their motor and communication skills continue to develop. Their speech will progress to several words, but tantrums may start to appear as they become easily frustrated. Walking will improve to running and climbing, and injuries are common as they explore their surroundings and push the limits of what they have tried. They may resist discipline, and these confrontations over the coming months may be the early signs of what some parents call the "terrible twos." Learning how to set boundaries and redirect your toddler will become important skills for you as a parent.

Before the Visit

Note any questions you have about communication skills, eye contact, pointing, signing, etc.

Questions for Today's Checkup

1.

2.

3.

Bring With You

- Diapers and wipes
- Acetaminophen or ibuprofen, if needed
- Healthy snack(s)
- Your list of questions
- Books or toys for the waiting or examination room (They are a must at this age. One-and-a-half-year-olds like to keep busy!)
- Hand wipes to keep your toddler clean as he wanders and explores his environment
- Forms required by child care facilities, if needed

During the Visit

➡ Your discussion today will focus largely on social and language development, best ways to maintain a healthy diet and healthy sleep habits, and planning for potty training.

➡ Expect a full set of measurements (ie, temperature, height, weight, and head circumference), as in the first few visits. Your doctor should discuss with you concerns on your list, review safety and child care, and fully examine your child. This is a good chance to mention any plans to return to work or school and discuss any concerns about child care options you may have.

➡ Developmental screening is recommended by the American Academy of Pediatrics at 9, 18, and 30 months of age.

➡ For this visit, the Centers for Disease Control and Prevention and the American Academy of Pediatrics recommend completing the hepatitis A series or starting it if not given yet, as well as any previously missed vaccines.

➡ If it is flu vaccine season (and it was not at the last checkup), is underway, the Centers for Disease Control and Prevention and the American Academy of Pediatrics also recommend an infant dose of flu vaccine; a repeat dose of flu vaccine will be needed if your child did not get 2 doses the previous flu season.

➡ Do not give acetaminophen in advance, which suppresses fever. Your doctor will want to know if your child has a fever at the checkup and may even delay vaccines if it is high.

After the Visit

☐ Schedule your 2-year visit and your follow-up flu vaccine if needed.

☐ Watch for your child to start climbing, and lower the crib to its lowest setting possible.

☐ Focus on speaking clearly and frequently to your toddler as you teach body parts, common objects, and animals and introduce colors and shapes.

☐ Your child's car seat should still be rear facing (read Car Seats on page 221 to understand when to change car seats).

Toddler Health Record: 18-Month Checkup

Toddler's Name:

Date:

Office:

Pediatrician Name:

Today's Weight: _____, which is the _____ percentile.

Today's Length: _____, which is the _____ percentile.

Today's Head Size: _____, which is the _____ percentile.

Feeding Habits:

Elimination Habits:

Sleep Habits:

Milestones Noted So Far:

Questions We Addressed:

1.

2.

3.

Things to Do After This Visit:

1.

2.

3.

Notes:

The 2-Year Checkup

Your child walks, jumps, and talks more at 2 years old, and the 2-year checkup is a time to gauge your toddler's progress according to his developmental and cognitive milestones.

Before the Visit

Note any concerns you have about your toddler's ability to communicate or walk. Review Is My Baby Sleeping Enough? When Will We Sleep Longer? on page 72 for information on sleep.

Questions for Today's Checkup

1.

2.

3.

Bring With You

- Diapers and wipes, as well as acetaminophen or ibuprofen (now that your toddler is older than 6 months) for use after today's immunizations
- Your list of questions and notes on communication, sleep, or both
- Forms required by child care facilities, if needed

During the Visit

→ Your discussion today will focus largely on communication and safety and may include referrals for hearing or speech evaluations if your child needs help with communication.

→ Expect a full set of measurements (ie, temperature, height, weight, and head circumference), as in the first visits. Your doctor should discuss with you concerns on your list, review safety and toddler care, and fully examine your toddler.

→ Ask your pediatrician about transitioning to lower-fat cow's milk and starting a daily vitamin.

→ Your toddler may have blood tested for lead and hemoglobin.

→ For this visit, the Centers for Disease Control and Prevention and the American Academy of Pediatrics recommend completing the hepatitis A vaccine series, as well as any previously missed vaccines.

➡ If flu vaccine season is underway, the Centers for Disease Control and Prevention and the American Academy of Pediatrics also recommend an infant dose of flu vaccine, with a repeat infant dose at least 1 month later if your child didn't receive 2 doses in the previous flu season.

➡ Don't give acetaminophen in advance, which suppresses fever. Your doctor will want to know if your child has a fever at the checkup and may even delay vaccines if it is high.

After the Visit

☐ Read Car Seats on page 221 for this age.

☐ Point out various things around you when running errands with your toddler. Even simple words such as *trucks*, *cars*, and *trees* provide an opportunity for your toddler to learn.

☐ Anticipate the desire for more independence and, with that, the typical tantrums of a 2-year-old. Do your best to praise him when he's acting well.

☐ Continue your toddler's nutrition as before.

☐ Read other books from the American Academy of Pediatrics to continue to educate yourself about toddlerhood, behavior, and beyond.

Toddler Health Record: 2-Year Checkup

Toddler's Name:

Date:
Office:
Pediatrician Name:

Today's Weight: _____, which is the _____ percentile.
Today's Length: _____, which is the _____ percentile.
Today's Head Size: _____, which is the _____ percentile.

Feeding Habits:

Elimination Habits:

Sleep Habits:

Milestones Noted So Far:

Questions We Addressed:

1.

2.

3.

Things to Do After This Visit:

1.

2.

3.

Notes:

Part 4

"What if My Baby Has...?"

Top 10 Concerns Parents Bring to the Office

Introduction: When Do I Call the Doctor?

Simply put, you should call your doctor any time you have a question or concern about your baby or toddler for which you'd like more information than a family member or friend can provide. As your parenting experience grows, you'll find that you can answer more questions yourself. You'll be able to determine what warrants a 3:00 am call. Knowing that your doctor has on-call nurses or staff to help in the middle of night with any question is helpful, but serious issues should get your doctor's attention.

When we think about problems that worry us as parents, they involve an infection (such as fever or breathing trouble) or our child's eating, drinking, sleeping, or pooping habits. You should consider calling your doctor's office when your child is not eating or drinking enough to urinate at least 4 times a day. Also, you should contact your doctor or seek medical attention for breathing distress, which includes poor color around the mouth or the ribs jutting out with rapid breathing. Babies cry for many reasons, and generally a mom or a dad can console a little one with a hug, feeding, or diaper change. If you can't console your little one, call your pediatrician's office for further help.

The point of Part 4 is to give you a starting point and some basic information for the most common symptoms you will face. Some things can be managed at home, but at some point illnesses should be evaluated and treated by a doctor. The next few chapters will help you decide when to seek medical care.

For the mobile-savvy parent, the American Academy of Pediatrics has a fantastic app called KidsDoc, which will guide you step-by-step through a multitude of symptoms, including when you should seek emergency department care.

Remember: No book should replace your primary care pediatrician. Consult your pediatrician with any questions or concerns if ever in doubt.

Constipation

👶 What is Constipation?

Constipation is defined as a decrease in frequency in stools or an increase in firmness to the point that they are difficult to pass. Decreased frequency of stools is actually common in breast-fed infants. While formula-fed infants usually pass stools 2 to 3 times a day, a breastfed infant may go several days between stools. As long as infants are eating well, passing gas, and not too fussy, such infrequent passing is likely not cause for concern.

Increased firmness in stools is what usually causes parents to seek treatment. Sometimes they can look like hard pellets, and sometimes they can be large. If your baby seems to have difficulty passing stools because they are too hard, you should contact your doctor. Also, do so if your baby has bleeding along with firm stools.

👶 What Isn't Constipation?

Newborns, during the first few weeks of life, often look like they struggle when they pass stools. Their faces may turn red, their bodies may shake, and every muscle in their bodies may seem to tighten up. If the stools that come out are soft, and newborns are passing stools a couple times a day, they are learning to poop and are not constipated. Imagine how you would look trying to pass stools while lying on your back instead of sitting up with the help of gravity as you do now.

🩲 What Can I Do for Firm Stools?

If stools are hard for your baby to pass because they are too firm, here are a few ideas that may work.

- For older than 1 month, juice may help. Prune, apple, or pear juices seem to work best (because they have the highest sugar content). Check with your doctor, but usually 1 to 2 ounces, once a day, is a safe starting point.
- Corn syrup may also be recommended by your doctor (light or dark work the same).
- If your baby has started spoon feeding, increasing fruits in his diet may help.
- Over-the-counter laxatives are marketed for babies, but you should check with your pediatrician before starting these.

Coughs and Colds

🍶 What Are Symptoms of a Cold?

Yellow or green mucus is common with a cold; people once thought those colors guaranteed a bacterial infection and required antibiotics, but now we know most green mucus may be just another sign of simple viral colds or allergies. A fever is also common. However, signs of labored breathing (eg, fast breathing, blue or pale color around the lips, audible wheezing, ribs or collarbones poking out, or nasal flaring with breathing) or signs of dehydration (eg, not drinking, few wet diapers, or few tears when crying) *are* a big deal and need to be seen immediately.

🍶 How Can I Treat My Baby's Cold Symptoms?

Stuffy Nose
For a stuffy nose, you can place a few drops of saline (salt water) into the nose to help thin the mucus and use a bulb

syringe to suction the mucus out. Running a cool-mist humidifier at the bedside helps humidify the air and keep nasal passages open. Also, drinking fluids to stay hydrated helps keeps secretions thin.

Fever

For a fever, acetaminophen or ibuprofen can be used based on age and weight; see Fever on page 163.

Cough

For a cough, honey is shown to be effective (*never give honey to a baby younger than 1 year*). Simple dosing is about 2.5 mL (half teaspoon) for ages 2 to 5 years and about 5 mL (one teaspoon) for ages 6 to 11 years.

What About Cough Medicines?

Cough medicines for kids were once easy to find on shelves in pharmacies. The American Academy of Pediatrics recommends over-the-counter cold medicines not be given to children younger than 2 years, as the side effects outweigh possible benefits. Over-the-counter cough and cold medicines are safe for use in children older than 6; use younger than this age should be only under supervision of a doctor.

⬛ What Is RSV?

The RSV germ (respiratory syncytial virus) is quick to spread from the nose and throat to the lungs of young infants and is a common cause of hospitalization. The illness this germ causes, called bronchiolitis, often starts like a simple stuffy nose but continues to worsen, causing labored breathing and dehydration that can peak around the fourth or fifth day. If your child was born premature, the risks of this illness are even higher, so a cold that seems to persistently worsen should prompt an evaluation. For more information on RSV, see Diagnosis: RSV on page 205.

⬛ What Is Pneumonia?

The term *pneumonia* applies to an infection within the lungs. It usually will cause fever, labored breathing, and chest pain or tightness. When symptoms are this severe, don't stay at home—get them checked out. Several bacteria, including whooping cough and many viruses, can cause this type of infection, and all require treatment.

Diaper Rashes

Chances are pretty good that your baby will, at some point, get a diaper rash. It doesn't mean you're doing a poor job of cleaning the diapers quickly enough; it just happens. The combination of an extremely moist environment under the diaper, along with the irritation caused by urine and stools, makes the skin break down (and even get infected) from time to time. The best prevention for diaper rashes is diaper changing as soon as possible after it becomes soiled. Most diaper rashes can be monitored at home, but some need to be seen by a pediatrician.

Here are 4 basic features we look for when checking out a diaper rash. If you have questions with any of these on your baby (especially yeast and bacterial infections), see your pediatrician.

Mild irritation. Most diaper rashes are no more than irritated skin. This will look like pink, flat skin marks in the diaper area. The best approach to treat these is to use a thick zinc oxide–based cream. Many of these creams are available over-the-counter.

Skin breakdown. Sometimes rashes get severe enough that the epidermis (protective outer skin) breaks down and your baby has painful rough exposed areas of skin underneath, often with a circular border. For these, zinc oxide–based creams are still helpful, but your doctor may recommend an over-the-counter liquid antacid to apply to the skin as well. These help cut the acidity of stools or urine and are soothing to the exposed wound.

Yeast infections. *Candida albicans* is a common yeast that causes infection under the diaper. It becomes a problem for a variety of reasons, especially when a baby is on an antibiotic, as healthy bacteria of the skin can be reduced, thus creating an ideal environment for yeast to grow. This rash will look more like pink-to-reddish dots, which form in clusters. It often starts near the rectum, or in groin creases, and works its way outward. For this rash, you will need an antifungal cream. Many pediatricians will call this in over the phone, and over-the-counter kinds are available. Some prescription antifungal creams may include a steroid component as well. In some cases, the steroid works as an anti-inflammatory but can mask more serious rashes and should not be used for more than 1 to 2 weeks. You will want to use antifungal cream until the rash is gone and 2 more days after that. If the rash doesn't improve in a few days, get it seen by your pediatrician.

🔗 **Bacterial infections.** One of the less common but more serious diaper rashes is caused by the bacteria *Staphylococcus aureus,* including methicillin-resistant *S aureus.* This will look like small pus bumps or pimples on a flat pinkish or red base, usually across the middle of the buttocks (away from the creases). These can be quite tender to the touch, and your baby will often seem uncomfortable. If your baby seems to have lesions that look as if they have pus coming out, and he has a fever or is otherwise uncomfortable, have him seen by your pediatrician within 24 hours.

Diarrhea

Diarrhea is a likely occurrence for your baby, usually at the most inopportune moment, and it's good to know why it happens and what to do about it.

✒ What Is Diarrhea?

First of all, all loose stools are not diarrhea. Breastfed babies may have up to 10 liquid, yellow, seedy stools a day, which are not considered to be diarrhea. In a few months, those babies may only produce stools once every few days, and that's fine too. You can expect a wide range of elimination by babies, and—as long as they're thriving, have no fever or vomiting, feed well, and gain weight—just going with the flow is okay. In many cases, frequent stools may make you initially think that your baby has a stomach virus or that her digestion is off track (which could be from an unusual food, excess juice, or salivation from ongoing teething). When she is acting well but having frequent liquid stools, we say she has mild diarrhea.

✐ What Can I Do for My Baby's Diarrhea?

Your goal when your baby has diarrhea should be to help keep her hydrated while her immune system clears the virus. Continue to breastfeed as often as your baby would like, or allow your baby to continue drinking her formula, or her usual diet, as long as she prefers. Interestingly, only a few kids (less than 10%) develop temporary lactose intolerance during a mild stomach virus, and the rest actually get better faster if you "feed through" the diarrhea. Many people ask about electrolyte solutions for babies. Those that are specifically designed for children have a balance of sugars and salts that can especially help an older child with diarrhea and dehydration, but for babies, discuss electrolyte solutions with your doctor first. Sports drinks and juices are far too sugary and can worsen a baby's diarrhea.

✐ What Kinds of Infections Cause Diarrhea?

Not all stomach or intestinal infections are from common viruses. Some bacterial infections (especially those caused by *Salmonella* species and *Escherichia coli*) and parasites also start with diarrhea and may progress to include blood in the stools, cramping pain, and fever. Babies with these symptoms need to be examined by a pediatrician.

Regardless of the number of stools, babies who have less than 6 wet diapers per day, who have abdominal pain or frequent vomiting, or who are not making tears when crying may be dehydrated and need to be seen by their pediatrician.

Falls and Head Trauma

🚲 What Signs Should I Look For?

For some warning signs of head trauma, you should seek immediate medical attention. These may happen at the time of the injury or even hours after the injury. They include from least to most concerning

- Losing consciousness
- Vomiting
- Acting more drowsy than usual
- Appearing especially fussy or confused
- Having drainage from the nose, ears, or eyes (This may be bloody or may be clear.)

In babies younger than 2 years, determining when an injury is mild, and when it is more serious, is not as easy for a parent. Seeking medical attention immediately is always the best course of action.

In addition, injuries can happen to more than just the head. One of the more common mistakes after a head injury is to look at only the head and ignore the rest of the body. Gently check the rest of your baby for bruises, lumps, or anything that looks different on one side of the body than the other. If your baby seems to not be moving an arm or leg as much as the other, or has pain when you try to move it, seek medical attention.

Where Should I Take My Baby for Evaluation?

For a head injury in a baby, evaluation in an emergency department is best. It is open 24 hours a day, has immediate access to an x-ray department if imaging is needed, and, in severe cases, has access to a neurologist or other trauma specialist. If you are second-guessing whether you should go to the emergency department, at least contact your pediatrician's office and have your baby seen. In the evening, your pediatrician's office should have an after-hours line to call for advice if you're not sure. Either way, if you are on the fence about whether to watch or take in, this is one case for which being cautious is a good idea. Even if your pediatrician determines your baby is healthy and not needing a computed tomography scan, having the injury checked out is often worth the peace of mind.

🚲 Do I Need to Keep My Baby Awake After a Head Injury?

Whether to keep a baby awake after a head injury is a common question. Always check with your doctor first, but, in most cases, sleep as usual is allowed. Your doctor may want you to see if your baby arouses every few hours or so the first day.

Fever

What Is a Fever?

A fever is when the body's baseline temperature is higher than expected, usually in response to an infection or other illness. While many parents consider anything higher than 98.6°F (37°C) to be a fever, most doctors consider a fever when the temperature hits 100.4°F (38°C) or higher. Some parents and doctors use the general term *low-grade fever* for temperatures between 98.6°F and 100.4°F, but this is more slang than science. Fever starts at 100.4°F or higher.

Do I Have to Treat a Fever?

You do not need to treat a fever every time, no. If your child has a fever and is not uncomfortable or fussy, nothing needs to be done. A fever is your body doing its job. If your child gets fussy, you may want to consider fever medicine to make him feel better, however. And remember, a fever is not an illness; it's the body's response to an illness. So even if medicine is reducing a fever, the illness that was causing the fever may still need to be evaluated.

How High of a Temperature Is Dangerous?

The height of a fever is less important than how your baby is acting. A baby who looks tired with a high temperature, but looks happier when the fever comes down, is less worrisome than one with a lower temperature whose color is poor or who is having difficulty staying alert, feeding, or breathing.

Any baby younger than 2 months with a fever of 100.4°F (38°C) or higher should receive medical attention immediately. For any child older than 2 months, at any point, if the fever is high enough that you are uncomfortable (as most parents would be if their baby's temperature were higher than 105°F [40.5°C]), please contact your pediatrician.

Only high temperatures caused by *external* heat are dangerous by themselves. This is called hyperthermia and is different than a fever, in which the body causes high temperatures internally.

Which Is Better: Acetaminophen or Ibuprofen? Can I Alternate Them?

No clear evidence suggests that of acetaminophen or ibuprofen, one is safer or more effective in treating a simple fever. Alternating between acetaminophen and ibuprofen can increase the chance of medication error, so it is generally discouraged.

Always check with your pediatrician before changing dosage or using a combination of fever-reducing medications.

Should I Give Fever Medicines Before My Child Receives Vaccines?

No, we do not recommend giving fever medicines before immunizations. A recent study shows that pretreatment could reduce the immune response that comes from the immunization. Your pediatrician should know if your baby or toddler has a fever on the day you come in for vaccines, and pretreating could mask it. Also, limited evidence suggests that giving fever medicines reduces pain or discomfort associated from getting shots.

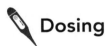

Dosing

Acetaminophen

For the acetaminophen described in Table 4-1, the concentration will be 160 mg/5 mL, and the package will usually be labeled "infants'" or "children's." *This can be given up to every 4 hours (but no more than 5 times in a 24-hour period).* Dosage should ideally be based on your child's weight and not his age. Always use the dosing device that comes with the medicine or that your doctor or pharmacist tells you to use. Never use teaspoons, tablespoons, or other household spoons to measure medicine.

Table 4-1 Dosing of Acetaminophen for Babies and Toddlers Based on Weight

Weight, pounds	Dose, mL
6–11	1.25
12–17	2.5 (or ½ teaspoon)
18–23	3.75
24–35	5.00 (or 1 teaspoon)

Ibuprofen

The ibuprofen described in Table 4-2 is the 50 mg/1.25 mL "infant concentrated drops" version. Ibuprofen liquid comes in a children's version as well, which is *less* concentrated (ie, 100 mg/5 mL). The infants' should come with a dropper; if, instead, it comes with a small cup or spoon, double check that it isn't the children's. Always use the dosing device that comes with the medicine or that your doctor or pharmacist tells you to use. Never use teaspoons, tablespoons, or other household spoons to measure medicine. *Infant drops can be given up to every 6 hours (no more than 4 times in a 24-hour period), starting at 6 months, or younger, if instructed by your doctor.*

Table 4-2 Dosing of Ibuprofen for Babies and Toddlers Based on Weight

Weight, pounds	Dose, mL
12–17	1.25
18–23	1.875
24–35	2.5 (or ½ teaspoon)

Flat Spot on the Head

Because of the birthing process, a newborn's head often appears less round than parents expect. Some come out cone shaped; others, lopsided. Pediatricians sometimes joke that this is the real reason we put hats on newborns in the nursery—to hide their head shape. Different shapes happen because a newborn's skull is not a solid bone like in adults; it's made up of several bony plates that are not fused together. You will feel a ridge (called a suture line) where any 2 plates meet. Where all suture lines meet on top of the head is the "soft spot," called the fontanel. Unusual head shapes we see from birthing generally correct on their own by 4 to 8 weeks of age.

Why Does the Back of My Baby's Head Still Have a Flat Spot?

After 2 months, some infants continue to have a flat spot on the back of their head. This is often the result of infants sleeping on their backs. While sudden infant death syndrome has decreased significantly since the Safe to Sleep campaign (an expansion of the Back to Sleep campaign) was introduced, it has led to an increase in flat spots. The medical diagnosis is called positional plagiocephaly, and it's caused by pressure of sleeping in one head position for an extended period of time (an infant's skull and bones are moldable). Also, a small stripe of baldness may form where the head lies against the mattress. Positional plagiocephaly is temporary, benign, and does not lead to other medical or neurologic issues. The head will round out over the next few months, and the hair will grow back as well. In fact, your doctor may compliment you if she notices a flat spot on the back of the head because it means you are doing a good job of having your baby sleep on his back.

What if the Flat Spot Is Somewhere Other Than the Back of the Head?

Not all flat spots on the back of the head are positional plagiocephaly. Other forms of plagiocephaly are less symmetric (ie, one side of the head is shaped differently than the other). Asymmetric plagiocephaly is usually believed to be a result of increased time in a lopsided position while in the womb and usually cannot be prevented. Your pediatrician may notice this at the 2-month checkup, or it may not get pronounced until the 4-month checkup. This form of plagiocephaly also does not lead to neurologic issues but often results in the need for some corrective action. One reason to correct asymmetric plagiocephaly is because it can lead to, or be worsened by, torticollis, in which uneven neck muscle tightness causes the head to be held at a tilt. To correct this, your doctor may recommend head positioning and neck-stretching exercises or may refer you to a pediatric physical therapist. If it progresses further, some pediatricians will treat it with a cranial orthotic molding helmet. This is a custom-fitted helmet to apply mild pressure in the right areas to correct any head asymmetry. It is not painful for your baby and is usually worn for several months, depending on severity of the correction needed.

Could This Be Anything Else?

Yes, not all head asymmetry is plagiocephaly. One other cause is craniosynostosis, which means the head sutures close too quickly. This can generally be detected by a pediatrician during well-child visits and is not something a parent should have to figure out on his own. Craniosynostosis can lead to severe head-shape issues and can restrict brain growth. Diagnosis is ultimately made by imaging and treated by a neurosurgeon to surgically reopen the sutures. This is a rare condition, but if your infant's head shape concerns you, and you don't have a checkup scheduled for the near future, make an appointment.

Teething

Teething can be harder on some babies than others. The good news is that most babies will get through teething without requiring any medical care. The first teeth often become visible through the gums at about 6 or 7 months of age, and these are usually the bottom front incisors. However, for several months leading up to this, the teeth buds are growing within the gums. Also, many babies' teeth will come in before or after the expected age, and in most cases this does not suggest a problem.

What Are the Most Common Symptoms of Teething?

- Fussiness
- Drooling, in some cases severe enough to go through multiple shirts a day
- Chewing more frequently on everything (eg, hands, toys)

Can Teething Cause Fever, Cold Symptoms, or Diarrhea?

Because older kids and teenagers all get their adult teeth without fever, cold symptoms, or diarrhea, many experts believe these symptoms stem not from teething but from the fact that a baby is more likely to have his hands in his mouth after touching everything around him, making him more prone to catching various minor viral infections that cause fever, cold symptoms, and diarrhea.

How Can We Treat Teething?

Treatment of teething depends on a baby's level of discomfort. Many babies don't require any treatment, but a few options include

- **Acetaminophen** (eg, Tylenol) may help as a fever- and pain-reducer for the baby. If the baby is older than 6 months, ibuprofen (eg, Motrin or Advil) can be used, but discuss this with your pediatrician.
- **Just about anything that can massage the gums,** such as an infant toothbrush or a terrycloth washcloth, can be useful.

- **Cool teething rings.** Be sure not to use frozen rings for longer than 5 to 10 minutes, as the cold can cause frostbite to the gums.
- **Teething biscuits** are types of food that are made to give relief to the gums but still dissolve for easy digestion when the baby has no teeth to grind.

Avoid herbal teething tablets that are available in some pharmacies or herbal stores. These often contain ingredients that cause concern in many pediatricians, including belladonna and caffeine. Teething tablets are also a choking hazard.

Thrush

What Is Thrush?

Thrush is a yeast infection of the mouth caused by an organism known as *Candida albicans. C albicans* can appear in anyone with an immature or weakened immune system, so babies over the first few months of life are easy targets. Thrush can also appear as a result of some medications, especially antibiotics and "breathing treatments" (ie, medications used for wheezing). If your baby is taking a liquid antibiotic, rinsing her mouth with water after giving her medicine can help decrease the risk of thrush.

What Does It Look Like?

Thrush is one of the most common benign infections that can occur during the newborn period. It shows up as a white, bumpy, cottage cheese–like substance inside the mouth. It is usually found inside the cheeks, inside the lips, or across the roof of the mouth.

Often thrush can be suspected in a baby with a white tongue. If a baby has a minimally white top of the tongue, she may just have residual breast (human) milk or formula on it.

The best way to find out is to take a clean finger or another firm object and gently scrape the tongue. If a white substance comes right off, and is only on the tongue, it is probably not thrush and does not need to be treated. Also, thrush will usually spread around the mouth to inside the lips and cheeks within just 1 or 2 days, so if the tongue has been white for several days but the rest of the mouth is clear, it's less likely to be thrush as well.

What Are the Complications?

Thrush can cause discomfort for a baby, and decreased feeding, and even lead to breast pain for a mother if spread to her during breastfeeding by direct contact. If this happens, the mother should call her obstetrician-gynecologist for treatment. But in most cases mothers will still be able to breastfeed.

How Does Thrush Get Treated?

Usually a visit or a call to your doctor will lead to a prescription medication for thrush. (This is one of few medications many pediatricians will prescribe without office evaluation.) The medicine is a liquid that is applied 3 to 4 times a day to inside the mouth. This can be given by a dropper or syringe or applied with a Q-tip. The length of treatment may vary, but a good rule of thumb is to keep treating thrush 2 days past when the lesions seem to be gone.

Vomiting and Dehydration

Vomiting is the forceful ejection of the contents of the stomach and is a natural reflex the body has developed to rid itself of unhealthy substances.

Why Do Babies Vomit?

Most times your baby or toddler may be vomiting because of symptoms of a stomach virus, and these usually resolve in less than a day. They sometimes are accompanied by diarrhea and fever (see Diarrhea on page 157 and Fever on page 163 for tips on managing these symptoms), and all symptoms usually resolve within 3 to 5 days.

Other causes of vomiting can be more serious, so be sure to call your doctor if your baby has a fever, cannot hold down sips of clear fluids, is having continuous abdominal pain, or is showing signs of dehydration.

How Would I Recognize Dehydration?

Mild to moderate dehydration includes symptoms such as being less playful than usual, producing between 3 and 6 wet diapers per 24 hours, having less tears when crying, and having a sunken fontanel (flat spot) lying down.

Severe dehydration produces more fussiness, 1 or 2 wet diapers in a 24-hour period, unusual sleepiness, and cool, discolored, or wrinkled skin.

 # How Do I Prevent Dehydration in My Baby?

To prevent dehydration, small, frequent sips of an oral rehydration solution can be given safely at home for any infant older than 6 months with even mild signs of dehydration. Ask your pediatrician which solution he prefers. For babies younger than 6 months, your pediatrician should be contacted for possible evaluation. Water in quantities of more than a few sips can affect salt balance in a baby's body and should be avoided. Another common mistake is to give a large quantity of liquid to a baby who seems thirsty after throwing up. Give frequent, small amounts of liquids to avoid risk of more vomiting.

Can I Use Any Medications at Home to Help My Vomiting Baby or Toddler?

Effective medicines for vomiting are available for older babies and toddlers. However, most doctors won't prescribe these until after your child has been evaluated to make sure nothing more serious is going on. Also, you should not use medications from a prior prescription without having your child evaluated for the current problem.

 ## What if My Baby Seems to Spit Up a Small Amount of Breast Milk or Formula After Feedings?

Babies who spit up after feeding are not vomiting. Essentially, every baby refluxes a little milk back up the throat and out the nose or mouth. It's not a big concern if the baby is gaining weight, generally happy, and not choking or having trouble breathing. See Diagnosis: Gastroesophageal Reflux Disease on page 199 if you think this might be occurring.

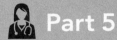 **Part 5**

A Doctor's Dozen

Top 12 Diagnoses Made in the Office

Diagnosis: Asthma

Asthma is the term used for the tendency to cough or wheeze after exposure to particular triggers such as exercise, colds, or allergies. Essentially, your child's immune system is over-reacting to common irritants; instead of just an expected, healthy cough to clear his throat, he has a persistent, exaggerated response (called an exacerbation) and can't breathe as he should for awhile afterward. If your child exhibits these signs, talk with your doctor. Tests may be able to find the specific trigger, and your child will need a thorough evaluation for other causes of cough and wheezing as well. Wheezing is *not* the same thing as congestion; it is a high-pitched whistling sound coming from the chest when a child exhales.

Diagnosis

If your doctor diagnoses asthma in your child, know that 3 things happen in your child's lungs when he starts to cough or wheeze.

1. Muscles lining the airways start to tighten, making them too narrow for air to easily flow.
2. Mucus is secreted that congests the chest.
3. Lining of the airways itself becomes swollen and inflamed, overreacting to whatever triggered the problem.

Medications and Treatment

Your pediatrician can prescribe medications for asthma to help manage the symptoms. Quick-relief medications, formerly known as "rescue medications," relieve some of the muscle constriction quickly and give fast relief from the wheezing and cough. More severe or persistent asthma may require controller medications (such as inhaled corticosteroids) to prevent mucus secretion or airway inflammation that worsens the symptoms as well. Controller medications need to be taken every day to be effective. Check with your health care professional for her recommended controller medication.

Some asthma medications can be inhaled from a nebulizer machine—an air compressor which pushes air through a medicine-filled cup, producing a cloud of inhalable medication—or from an inhaler, also called a "puffer," which is a little pressurized can of medicine, with a spacer—a tube to slow the pressurized stream of medicine so it can be inhaled correctly. Many people use their inhalers without spacers, but they don't work well that way, especially for children. Also, some asthma medications are given by mouth, including preventive medicines and medicines for acute flare-ups (such as oral steroids).

Living With Asthma

How you go about treating asthma depends on how severely or frequently problems flare up. If a trigger is obvious—for example, a cat triggering symptoms in an allergic child—the answer, unfortunately, might be to find a new home for the cat. Many times, a referral to a pediatric allergy/asthma specialist is the best way to identify triggers. If the trigger can't be found, or if it is one that can't be avoided (eg, cold air or exercise), the focus will be on reducing your child's symptoms and making him feel better. For kids who rarely have episodes when they cough or wheeze (less than twice a month), simply giving a quick-relief medication to use when needed may be enough (but check with your health care professional). For kids with frequent exacerbations (ie, either more than twice per week during the day or twice per month and waking them at night), they may need to take a controller medication every day to prevent themselves from having serious breathing problems that can lead to hospital or emergency department visits. Ask your doctor about how to best care for your child if it interferes with his daily routine.

Diagnosis: Colic

Colic can be one of the most frustrating problems for parents. Typically showing up at 3 or 4 weeks of age, this unexplained problem causes otherwise healthy babies to have prolonged crying episodes (up to 3 to 5 hours), usually later in the day, most days, until 3 to 4 months. Babies with colic often pass gas and straighten their legs or pull their legs in. No one knows exactly what causes colic, although immaturity of the intestinal tract may play a role. Immaturity of the nervous system, resulting in overstimulation, is the more likely cause.

When we see crying babies who might have colic, we consider two important questions.

Might Other Problems Besides Colic Explain the Crying?

- Reflux, or movement of acid and stomach contents into the esophagus, is often common but can cause pain or difficulty with breathing, in which case we call it gastroesophageal reflux disease (GERD). Babies with GERD may arch their back as they fuss and often spit up as many as 1 or 2 hours after feeding. If you have questions about whether GERD may be a problem for your baby, please talk with your pediatrician.

- Intolerance or allergy to a component of breast milk (such as dairy products in mom's diet) or formula can present with colic and can be accompanied by vomiting, dry and irritated skin rashes, or blood in the stools. If these symptoms occur, colic is not the only problem, and you should bring in your baby to be evaluated by your pediatrician. Your doctor may advise you to remove dairy from your diet if you're breastfeeding. If your baby is formula fed, your pediatrician may recommend a formula change. Ask your doctor which formula is recommended, and remember that it can take several days or longer to see improvement after a formula change.

- If your baby has a fever, diarrhea, or rash; is congested or coughing; or isn't eating well, colic is not her problem.

What Can Parents Do to Help Their Baby?

If you do not suspect the symptoms listed above, consider focusing on reducing your baby's discomfort.

- Swaddle your baby in a large thin blanket to help her feel snug.
- Hold your baby, and sway gently from side to side to help her find relief.
- Turn on soothing background or white noise.
- Try to avoid overfeeding your baby, and try to wait 2 hours before the start of consecutive feedings.
- If breastfeeding or formula feeding is well established, try a pacifier to help soothe your baby between feedings.
- While not recommended by the American Academy of Pediatrics, some parents try over-the-counter medicines containing simethicone, which are intended to prevent gas bubbles from forming. Other products include some herbal remedies to try to help with pain. Studies show that these products are not much more effective than placebo or sugar water, but some parents report that they do help. Recent studies have shown that probiotics may be effective in reducing colic symptoms.
- Sometimes bathing, or even taking a car ride (both for the parents' sanity and the baby to get a little vibration), can be helpful.

Typically, fussiness and colic increase until about 6 to 8 weeks of age, start to decrease, and are usually gone by 3 to 4 months. The good news about this condition is that it goes away on its own, is harmless, and causes no future problems for your baby.

Diagnosis: Cradle Cap

At some point, over the first few months, you may notice flakes or scales peeling at the top of your baby's head. The affected area may be a small patch, or it can be extensive. It is most likely seborrhea, more commonly known as cradle cap.

What Is Cradle Cap?

Cradle cap is neither an infection nor a fungus; it's simply peeling, flaking, oily skin, much like dandruff that adults get. The flakes may be white, yellow, or brownish and sometimes can have a foul smell to them. No one exactly knows why it happens, but it's not something you could have prevented. It does not hurt, is not contagious, and should not cause your baby to be fussy at all. Sometimes it can extend outside of the hair. You may notice flaking in the eyebrows, redness around the sideburns area, and even redness with cracking along the crease behind the ears.

How Is It Diagnosed?

Cradle cap is usually diagnosed at home by parents. If the treatment described next is not helping, or if you are concerned it could be something else, evaluation by your pediatrician is always a good idea.

 ## How Is It Treated?

The best treatment for cradle cap is to use an adult dandruff shampoo. The main ingredient, selenium sulfide, helps reduce the oiliness that causes cradle cap. Sometimes these shampoos can make the head tingle but should not hurt. A good approach is first to scrub the shampoo into the scalp for 2 to 3 minutes and then to rinse it out, repeating the process about every 2 days. Also, gentle brushing with a soft infant hairbrush may help. But don't pick at it too hard; you don't want to break the skin and possibly cause an infection.

Using baby oil for cradle cap makes the top of the head greasy so the flakes are no longer noticeable, but it does not take care of the problem. It's a start if it helps you gently brush out the flakes, but you'll need to follow it with the shampoo.

Diagnosis: Croup

 ## What Is Croup?

Croup is generally a seasonal respiratory illness, which usually shows up in fall and early winter and is most common in babies and children 6 months to 3 years of age. Croup is the sudden onset of a "barky" cough, often at night, and sometimes accompanied by a harsh, tight sound that comes from difficulty drawing air *in* after the cough. It is usually caused by a virus, the most common called parainfluenza virus (different from the flu).

 ## What Are the Signs?

The sound of croup is often described as a seal barking and comes from swelling in the airways. Often children with croup have a 1- or 2-day history of a runny nose and sometimes a fever when their barking cough begins. The cough of croup can occur for 2 to 4 nights in a row, but the child often appears better during the day.

How Is It Treated?

Treatment of mild croup includes simple home measures such as steaming up the bathroom and letting a child inhale the warm moist air, standing outside inhaling the cold air, or using a cool-mist humidifier to ease his breathing indoors. Other home remedies, such as cold medicines, do not help croup (and may worsen the condition if they prevent the child from coughing up mucus from infection). Antibiotics do not help, as the problem is a viral illness and antibiotics only help bacterial infections. Though these remedies may help some children, there are no studies that prove inhaling steam or moist, cool night air is effective.

 ## Do We Need to See a Doctor?

A mild cold with a slightly barky cough may not require medical attention. If your child is making a tight whistling sound when breathing in after the barking sound, has a bluish color around the mouth or fingernails, or seems to be struggling to breathe, croup may be more severe and you should take your child to the emergency department where some inhaled medications can help. If your child is older than 1 year, and does not appear to have difficulty breathing, visiting your pediatrician in the morning should be fine. The most common treatment by pediatricians for croup is a steroid medicine to reduce airway swelling, as a one-time injection or an by mouth.

As with any cold, croup can be accompanied by problems such as ear infections, sinus infections, or pneumonia, which you can discuss with your pediatrician.

Diagnosis: Ear Infection

If an ear infection has been diagnosed in your baby, she is not alone. This is one of the most common infections of infancy and is not always obvious because symptoms can vary.

 ## What Is an Ear Infection? Why Did It Happen?

We all make mucus in the deeper parts of our ears, and this naturally drains down our eustachian tubes to the back of our throats. Congested babies and toddlers can make too much mucus to drain down the eustachian tube, so that mucus sits in the little space deep in our ears called the middle ears and becomes a breeding ground for an ear infection.

 ## Did It Happen From Bathwater or Pool Water Getting In?

Because an ear infection happens in the middle ear *behind* the eardrum, it has to come from the back of the nose and throat, not from outside the ear (such as from bathwater or pool water). On a related note, as long as the eardrum is intact, you cannot treat a middle ear infection with drops in the ear.

How Is It Diagnosed?

An ear infection can usually only be detected when your pediatrician looks at the eardrum through an otoscope. A healthy eardrum should be a pearly gray color, while an ear infection will often show a bulging eardrum with redness and fluid behind it.

What Symptoms Might Indicate an Ear Infection?

Generally, kids with an ear infection will have pain, and they won't sleep well at night. Seeing a child pulling at an ear while she plays is not usually enough to require a doctor visit, but ear pulling with recent cold or allergy symptoms, fever, and worsening pain and sleep should be checked out. There is no shame in going to the doctor only to find out the ears are fine.

How Are Ear Infections Treated?

Younger Than 6 Months

Babies younger than 6 months are more prone to problems if an ear infection spreads or worsens, so essentially all those in this early age group require antibiotics by mouth or by injection for ear infection treatment.

From 6 Months Through 24 Months

For the last few decades, almost all children with ear infections, regardless of age, were treated with antibiotics. However, pediatricians and parents are slowly becoming more comfortable with observing ear infections without always prescribing antibiotics, but this is only in cases when the child is old enough for the risk of invasive infections to be low, when pain is controllable with ibuprofen or acetaminophen, and when no fever, or just a low fever, is present.

If your child is in significant pain, shows signs of spreading infection, or has a high fever, she will need an oral antibiotic to treat her ear infection.

If your doctor diagnoses and treats an ear infection, he will usually schedule a follow-up appointment in about 4 to 6 weeks. We don't schedule it too soon because even if the antibiotic is finished and the infection is killed, the fluid can take a little longer to finish clearing out of the ear, so the ear may not look completely healthy after only 10 days. You should keep this appointment regardless; just because your child is not fussy anymore does not mean the infection fully went away, and it is best to be certain that no fluid remains behind the ear to interfere with hearing or lead to another infection.

Do We Need to See an ENT Specialist?

An ear infection that won't resolve after several treatments usually means a child has an eustachian tube that is not working like it should. After several ear infections too close together (most pediatricians wait for 4 to 6 infections over 6 months), it may be time for a referral to an ear-nose-throat (ENT) specialist, and your pediatrician will help you decide when to take this route. While we wait for the child's eustachian tube to slowly grow larger and reduce ear infection tendencies, an ENT specialist may place a small plastic tube through the eardrum to allow the middle ear to stay ventilated. This may improve hearing during a critical time of speech development, although researchers are still looking at the effects of tube placement on speech.

Diagnosis: Eczema

Many babies develop dry skin during infancy, but some babies are prone to a skin condition called eczema (or atopic dermatitis). More than just dry skin, the skin of someone with eczema is itchy, red, irritated and sometimes becomes moist, thickened, or crusted.

How Does My Baby or Toddler Get a Diagnosis of Eczema?

You'll need to bring your baby or toddler to your pediatrician to have eczema diagnosed, and it is usually diagnosed by history and examination alone. Allergy, skin, or blood testing might be considered if the eczema does not respond to standard treatments or if your doctor thinks the eczema is being flared up by food or environmental allergies.

Is It Common? Why Did My Child Develop Eczema?

Eczema is one of the most common skin conditions seen by pediatricians and dermatologists and appears to have a genetic basis, running in families along with asthma and nasal allergies. Sometimes eczema can be triggered by foods or allergens (such as animals or specific plants), but in many cases it starts without an obvious cause.

 # What Do I Need to Watch For?

In addition to red, irritated, and dry skin, untreated eczema can lead to skin bacterial infections (producing a yellow crusty discharge) or viral infections (often with wart-like growths). Contact your doctor if you suspect that your child's eczema is getting worse.

 # What Can I Do to Help My Child?

- Moisturize your child's skin twice a day and immediately after baths.
- Don't use hot water or much soap when bathing your child, as over-washing can cause eczema to worsen.
- Avoid irritants by using mild soaps and hypoallergenic detergents, and skip fabric softener in the dryer.
- Help your child stop scratching by covering affected areas and keeping his hands distracted with other things, such as toys, because itching can irritate the skin and worsen the rash.

- If you know your child is allergic to something in the environment (such as grass outside or a cat inside), avoid contact as much as you can.

Medications can help eczema, but since this book covers material for children up to 2 years old, we encourage you to talk with your doctor before using medicines such as antihistamines, steroid creams, and ointments.

Will My Child Have Eczema His Whole Life?

Fortunately, most eczema gets better by the time a child is 4 years old, but some people continue to have eczema during their life. The good news is that many effective treatments exist and can improve the itching and irritation, as well as appearance of the skin.

Diagnosis: Gastroesophageal Reflux Disease

It's perfectly normal for otherwise healthy babies to reflux, or spit up, during infancy. The muscles that tighten the lower esophagus near the stomach, called the lower esophageal sphincter, often have not become strong enough to keep stomach contents (ie, breast milk, formula, and stomach acid) in the right place. Spitting up is commonly a simple yet messy event and is more of a laundry problem than a medical one. The usual reasons for spitting up include slight overfeeding or playing after feeding, or sometimes it occurs for no reason at all. Occasional spitting up in an otherwise well baby usually does not require medical care.

Some babies, however, spit up to the point when it *does* become a medical problem and may receive a diagnosis of gastroesophageal reflux disease (GERD, also called reflux) from their pediatrician. Babies with GERD usually have other symptoms, such as fussiness, poor weight gain, difficulty feeding, or repeated respiratory infections. There is no quick laboratory test for GERD. Sometimes special imaging procedures (eg, barium swallow or ultrasound) are necessary to rule out other conditions, but GERD is usually diagnosed by describing your baby's condition to your pediatrician during an office visit.

Gastroesophageal reflux disease usually gets better with some combination of the following 4 approaches and can differ by age:

Upright Positioning

Babies are often fussier when they lie flat but feel relief when they lie with their head upright at about a 30° to 40° angle. Try to keep your baby upright after feedings for at least 45 minutes.

Thickened Feedings

In older babies (usually older than 4 to 6 months), rice cereal is sometimes added to breast milk or formula to thicken its consistency and minimize reflux. Most older babies are still able to take the mixture through the bottle but may need a nipple with a larger hole (such as a heavy-flow nipple). Some experts disagree about how effective this is, so talk with your pediatrician before thickening your baby's feedings.

Hypoallergenic Formulas

If your pediatrician feels a food allergy is contributing to reflux, she may switch your baby to a hypoallergenic formula. In all honesty, these can be expensive, but most babies outgrow reflux by 6 to 8 months and can often be switched back to less expensive standard formula.

Medications

If your baby's condition gets worse, with more discomfort or difficulty feeding, it is time to make an additional appointment to see your pediatrician and discuss whether further tests or treatments are required.

Diagnosis: Jaundice

What Is Jaundice?

Because jaundice usually happens in the first few days of life, this condition may be your introduction to health care for your baby. In short, jaundice is the yellow color many newborns' skin and eyes turn because of a chemical called bilirubin. Many babies get jaundice, and almost all cases resolve in the first few weeks of life.

Why Does It Happen?

As soon as your little bundle is born, he takes a big breath, and his body realizes that the extra red blood cells he was born with are no longer required. The spleen and liver start breaking down the extra blood cells so that the blood can get thinner and easier to pump. One of the side effects of this breakdown is the chemical bilirubin, which is what causes the yellow appearance characteristic of jaundice and most evident in the whites of the eyes and in the skin. The level of jaundice is usually measured by a blood test. Because red blood cell breakdown is required in a baby's blood, some level of jaundice is expected in all babies.

Jaundice can be more pronounced if a mom's blood type and baby's blood type are different. In some cases, a test called the Coomb's test is performed on the newborn's blood to check for reaction to mom's blood antibodies. Other problems that can intensify jaundice include prematurity, bruising from the birthing process, and even infection.

Is Jaundice Harmful?

Most jaundice isn't harmful, even though the level of bilirubin increases during the first few days of life. Pediatricians use a special chart—the bilirubin nomogram—to check the level of jaundice and compare it to expected levels based on a baby's age. Based on this chart, your doctor will let you know if the level is safe to watch or needs additional treatment. In extremely rare cases, if the level reaches the highest parts of the curve, the baby is at risk of nerve injury, called kernicterus. Thus, we start therapy well before these levels to avoid this injury.

How Is It Treated?

The most common therapy for jaundice is called phototherapy. This involves a machine (either an overhead light or a blanket with lights in it) that provides a certain level of UV light to be shined on your baby's skin. A nurse will show you how to do this, but generally your baby is naked except for a diaper and, in some cases, a mask for the eyes. Phototherapy may happen while your baby is in the hospital but is also common in the home setting. Once a baby is on phototherapy, repeated bilirubin levels are checked until the level reaches a point that the lights can be stopped. In the most severe jaundice cases, if the level gets too high, a transfusion may be required to quickly reduce it. This is usually done by a neonatologist.

Does Jaundice Come Back?

Once jaundice has started going away, it should not return. If, however, your baby appears yellow beyond the first 1 or 2 weeks, be sure to check with your doctor.

Diagnosis: RSV

What Is RSV?

Coughs and colds during a baby's first 2 years have many causes, but one of the viruses that typically appears between October and March is called RSV. This stands for respiratory syncytial virus. The virus can cause a wide range of symptoms, which can be worse for premature babies. In mild cases, it can look like a common cold with only a tolerable runny nose and fever. In severe cases, however, it can cause respiratory distress, including irritation of the large airway (ie, a "barky" cough called croup; see Diagnosis: Croup on page 189), or increased fluid and inflammation of the lungs, known as bronchiolitis, often diagnosed by a sound called a wheeze. During peak season, this contagious virus makes its way through schools and child care facilities by the spread of small droplets of mucus.

What Are the Symptoms of RSV?

Distinguishing RSV from a common cold is often difficult. The common cold usually has severe symptoms for 2 to 3 days and a mild resolution over a couple weeks. However, RSV can produce a more frothy runny nose, barky cough, or wheeze. Respiratory syncytial virus is also more likely to cause labored breathing, a need for extra oxygen, and susceptibility to bacterial infections such as ear infections and pneumonia.

 ## How Is RSV Diagnosed?

Your pediatrician may run a test in the office that diagnoses RSV by a nasal swab (similar to a Q-tip inserted into the nose). Because RSV does not become as severe in older children, the test is not run in all cases, usually just on infants and younger children. Also, the test is not 100% accurate, so it is only part of your doctor's evaluation in making the diagnosis.

 ## How Is It Treated?

Treatment for RSV involves addressing the symptoms. Because RSV is a virus, antibiotics do not play a role unless another infection presents as well. For mild cases, good hydration and nasal-bulb suction in babies may be all you need. We used to recommend cough medicines to suppress the cough, but in recent years studies have shown that these can cause more harm than good. Your pediatrician will decide if your child should have a medication prescribed. If wheezing is present, your pediatrician may start your child on breathing treatments. This is accomplished by a machine, called a nebulizer, which creates a cloud or steam of medicine that is inhaled. A child breathes this in for about 5 to 10 minutes, and it delivers the medicine directly to the lungs (similar to if you've seen someone with asthma use a "puffer" or inhaler). Noise and steam may seem scary to a child at first, but children quickly get used to it. Even when RSV seems to have passed the contagious period (usually 3 to 8 days but can be up to weeks), the symptoms may linger. If at any point you are not comfortable and feel that the illness is not getting better, definitely recheck with your pediatrician.

Does RSV Have a Vaccine?

There is no vaccine to prevent RSV. There is a monthly protein shot (palivizumab) that reduces the symptoms of RSV, but it is recommended only for babies that are at highest risk of hospitalization from RSV. This includes babies that were born 29 weeks premature or earlier or babies with certain chronic heart or lung diseases. Usually babies who should receive this shot are identified by newborn nursery staff before they go home, but if you have questions, check with your pediatrician.

Diagnosis: Strep Throat

 ## What Is Strep Throat?

Strep throat is when someone has a throat infection caused by specific bacteria called "strep" (or group A streptococci). It usually presents with fever and sore throat. Other typical symptoms include fussiness, swollen glands in the neck, and decreased appetite. Less common symptoms that can come with strep throat include abdominal pain or nasal discharge.

 ## How Is Strep Throat Diagnosed?

Your doctor will have a strong suspicion based on history and examination, but strep throat is best diagnosed with laboratory testing. Most pediatric offices can do a rapid strep test, which involves the throat being swabbed with a special cotton swab. Results are usually back in less than 10 minutes. Another test is a throat culture, which is obtained by the same special cotton swab and grown on a culture dish over 24 hours. The culture is slightly more accurate, so most office staff that do a rapid strep test will also do a throat culture if the rapid strep test is negative.

How Is It Treated?

Strep throat is a bacterial infection and can be treated with an antibiotic. The most common one used is amoxicillin by mouth for 10 days, but your doctor may use other options, including different antibiotics or even an antibiotic shot. It's important to finish the full course of the antibiotic, even if your baby feels better quickly. Strep throat that is not fully treated can lead to other problems, including abscess, rash (scarlet fever), heart issues (rheumatic fever), and kidney inflammation.

Are All Sore Throats Caused by Strep?

Many different viruses can cause the same symptoms as strep. Some that are seen in childhood include Coxsackie virus (the virus that causes hand-foot-mouth disease) and "mono." Some of these also cause a white-like discharge on the tonsils, so even this finding does not guarantee that strep is the cause of the infection. That's why doctors don't usually call in antibiotics for a sore throat but instead recommend you have your child evaluated. If the infection is caused by a virus, antibiotics will not be prescribed.

Diagnosis: Tear-Duct Obstruction

Nasolacrimal duct obstruction, or blocked tear duct, is a common newborn condition and eventually resolves on its own with time. Your newborn will have a watery drainage from one or both eyes. Sometimes the drainage gets crusty when your newborn's eyes are closed for sleeping, with the eye otherwise looking as it should.

How Do I Know if It's a Tear-Duct Obstruction or an Infection?

When the eye has a small amount of drainage, first get a clean wet washcloth and gently wipe the eye clean. Then see how the eye looks.

Check if

☐ The white of the eye is red or pink.
☐ Your baby has a fever.

☐ Your baby is not feeding well.

☐ Your baby is fussy.

☐ The eyelid looks red or swollen.

If your baby has any of the listed symptoms, the eye could be infected. For an eye infection, you should see your doctor that day.

However, if your baby has none of the listed symptoms (especially redness or swelling of the eye), she may have a blocked tear duct, in which case you can observe it at home, unless symptoms get worse.

How Do You Fix Tear-Duct Obstruction?

For persistent tear-duct obstruction, massage at the tear duct site may be attempted at home or recommended by your doctor (but is usually not required; it's controversial as to whether it helps). Gently massage over the hole in a circular motion with your index finger for about 1 minute, 3 times a day. Your pediatrician can show you how to do this, but wash your hands first, and make sure your nails are not too long. In rare cases, your pediatrician may refer you to a pediatric eye specialist if the drainage from the eye persists; referral usually occurs at around 9 to 12 months of age (or sooner for complications such as recurrent infection). Your doctor may then recommend probing of the tear duct, a simple procedure during which the canal is opened.

If you have any concern of infection, visit your doctor that day.

Diagnosis: Urinary Tract Infections

What Is a Urinary Tract Infection?

Naturally our urine is sterile and has no bacteria in it, but when bacteria enter urine and cause irritation of the kidneys, bladder, or connecting ducts, a urinary tract infection, often referred to as a UTI, occurs. Usually the bacteria come from the rectum or stools and enter through the urethra (ie, duct that connects the bladder to the outer vagina in girls or to the tip of the penis in boys). But the bacteria can enter from within the body as well. Different bacteria can be the cause, but the most common is *Escherichia coli,* which is found in the stools.

Who Gets a UTI?

Urinary tract infections occasionally occur in infancy and childhood and are more common for girls than boys. This is because of differences in anatomy; the urethra is shorter in girls, so bacteria have an easier time finding their way in from the outside.

About 3% of girls will get a UTI in infancy or childhood. About 1% of boys can get a UTI, but for a boy it's rare after the first year. Also, uncircumcised boys have a higher risk of UTI than circumcised boys in the first few months of life.

 ## What Are the Symptoms of a UTI?

In a baby, the only symptom may be fever and fussiness because babies cannot tell you where they are hurting. Also, urine may appear cloudy or foul smelling. A child old enough to tell you how she feels may report burning or pain with urination, a need to urinate more frequently, belly ache, or back pain. If it goes untreated, further symptoms can include loss of appetite and vomiting.

 ## How Is It Diagnosed?

The diagnosis of a UTI is made based on analysis of urine. Because a baby is not potty trained, urine is usually collected by a nurse, using a catheter to enter the urethra. Once urine is obtained, it can be quickly checked in most pediatric offices with a urine dipstick or urinalysis machine, which detects foreign substances in urine that may signify infection. Ultimately, a UTI is diagnosed by culture; the urine gets sent to a larger laboratory (typically a local hospital or national laboratory chain) to grow for the bacteria. Within 2 to 3 days, laboratory staff should be able to tell if bacteria is present, which bacterium it is (known as identification), and which antibiotics will work on this bacterium (known as sensitivities). Sometimes a complete blood count is checked along with urine studies. An elevated white blood cell count may indicate that the UTI is more severe, which may affect treatment decisions.

How Is a UTI Treated?

A UTI is treated with antibiotics. In most cases, an oral course is prescribed to last 7 to 14 days. If a baby appears especially ill, sometimes she is given an antibiotic shot first or even admitted to a hospital and given antibiotics through an IV until she improves. Even though urine culture may take 2 to 3 days to come back, a pediatrician usually begins antibiotics as soon as he has a high suspicion of infection. He will pick an antibiotic that has a high success rate with the most common bacteria causing UTIs. He can then change the antibiotic if the sensitivities show a better antibiotic choice or if the baby is not improving.

Part 6

On the Go Info

🔤 ABCs of Diaper Bag Must-haves

Too much to pack? We've got you started! Below is a list of must-pack items to take with you while traveling, as well as space to add your own items.

- ☐ Acetaminophen or ibuprofen
- ☐ Blanket
- ☐ Bibs
- ☐ Books
- ☐ Bottles
- ☐ Burp cloths
- ☐ Carrier or baby sling
- ☐ Changing pad
- ☐ Diaper cream
- ☐ Diapers (more than you think you will need)
- ☐ Diaper bag dispenser with bags (often comes in different colors!)
- ☐ Few toys
- ☐ Formula
- ☐ Gas drops
- ☐ Gallon-size bag or plastic bag for dirty clothes
- ☐ Hand sanitizer
- ☐ Nursing (breastfeeding) cover
- ☐ One more outfit than you think you'll need (Keep this in a plastic bag in case of any spills.)
- ☐ Pacifier (if using one)

- ☐ Paper towel, napkins, or tissue
- ☐ Pajamas if you are out later than bedtime
- ☐ Snacks (if old enough to get them)
- ☐ "Teethers"
- ☐ Thermometer
- ☐ Wipes
- ☐ _____
- ☐ _____
- ☐ _____

A travel notepad is included at the end of Part 6 that features space to list all important travel information and must-bring items for each of your traveling children.

Car Seats

Car seats are designed to reduce the likelihood of an injury to your child in the event of a car crash. Some of the most common questions we get are the following:

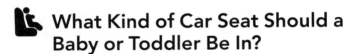 What Kind of Car Seat Should a Baby or Toddler Be In?

Babies should be in a rear-facing seat with a 5-point harness until they are at least 2 years of age (or if they have outgrown the maximum weight/height of their car seat). Parents usually start with an infant car seat and switch to a rear-facing convertible seat when their baby outgrows the size limit on the infant car seat. Some states still have laws in place that allow for turning around sooner than 2 years of age, but we, like the American Academy of Pediatrics, recommend parents follow the 2-year rule.

A child who is older than 2 or has outgrown the maximum weight/height of his rear-facing convertible seat can use a forward-facing car seat with a harness. He should stay in this until he passes the maximum weight/height allowed by the manufacturer.

How Do We Secure the Car Seat Properly?

Car seats should be placed in a frame that is already secured in the car by a seatbelt passing through the frame or by the LATCH (Lower Anchor and Tethers for Children) system. The rear-facing position is important enough to mention again; it protects a baby's head, neck, and spinal column better than the forward-facing position. If you have concerns about your car seat being properly secured, most cities have free car seat inspection options, including at hospitals and fire stations.

My Baby Seems Uncomfortable in His Rear-Facing Car Seat. Can I Turn It Around a Bit Earlier?

Many parents worry that their rear-facing baby is too cramped if his feet touch the back of the seat. This position may not seem optimal, but it is still a much safer alternative than turning forward too soon.

I Want to Keep My Baby Warm in the Car. Can She Wear Her Coat in the Car Seat?

You should take bulky coats and outer clothing off your baby before strapping into a car seat. The straps may feel snug at first, but a coat makes car seat straps fit less securely. If the weather outside is cold, you can lay the coat or a blanket on your baby and over the straps.

How Can I More Easily Fit My Baby in the Car Seat When We Leave the Hospital?

Usually, when mom and baby leave the hospital, mom leaves in a wheelchair and baby rides in her arms. It's a good idea to get the car seat up to the hospital room to check the fitting first. Car seat straps often need adjustment, and it's easier to do in the controlled environment of a hospital room than in a parking lot or parking deck.

If I'm Careful, Can I Take My Baby Out of the Car Seat for a Quick Feeding or Diaper Change?

At some point, you will take a road trip and be tempted to take your baby out of the car seat for a feeding or to change a diaper.

Maybe you are running late and want to get to your destination on time. *Never* take your baby out of the car seat when the car is moving. It's not about how good a driver you or your spouse is but more about the safety of your baby in a vehicle.

What Is the Best Car Seat Brand?

Car seats have no best brand, and a higher price does not always mean better. Definitely avoid used car seats, especially if you can't be sure of the history. Never use one if it has been in a car crash. Often times, damage to a car seat may not be discernible on the outside.

Travel Tips

Car Trips (Greater Than 2 Hours)

Birth to 2 Months

- Feed and burp your baby right before you leave to maximize the contented period after you start your trip.
- Anticipate stops every hour for diaper changes, feedings, and comforting and to adequately rest yourself.
- As long as your car is moving, your baby needs to be strapped in, so breastfeeding while driving is out. Bottle-feeding your baby while he's in the car seat creates a high potential for choking, so plan to stop frequently to soothe and feed your baby when needed.

At 2 to 12 Months

- During 2 to 12 months of age, babies sleep and feed more predictably and are more easily distracted, so you may have a better experience traveling.
- Stop frequently for diaper changes, and check often to see if your baby is uncomfortable or needs to be adjusted in his seat.

- Babies this age become observant and start watching the world go by but can become overstimulated and tire easily, so plan to stop for fresh air and stretching as the trip goes on.

At 12 to 24 Months

- Babies and toddlers around 12 to 24 months of age can be rambunctious, and sitting still can be difficult for them. Pack healthy snacks, books, stuffed animals, toys, games, and child-friendly music.
- Sing-alongs can be one of the easiest ways to soothe your child when he gets tired or cranky in the seat, and plan on time outside the car to run and play at rest stops to release their energy.

✈ Air Travel

Not-So-Commonly Known Basics

- Many airlines will let a child younger than 2 fly for free, but check with your preferred airline because this may not always guarantee you have a seat for your child if a ticket is not purchased. The safest air travel for a baby is to be strapped into a car seat in his own seat. This is the recommendation of both the Federal Aviation Administration and the American Academy of

Pediatrics. Some airlines offer reduced airfare for baby travelers. If you are using an infant car seat that can be installed without the base, this is usually all you need to take to install in an airplane seat, but not all car seats are approved for air travel, so check to see if yours is a government-approved child safety restraint system.

- Likewise, many airlines don't count baby-care items against your checked-bag limit, so you can check a car seat and a portable crib without paying extra fees. Verify your airline regulations to be sure.
- For international travel, remember that everyone, no matter how young, needs a passport. Just a birth certificate is not adequate to leave the country. A passport can take some time to process, so take care of it early if you anticipate a foreign trip in your baby's future.
- Timing is everything; anything to help your child sleep during travel will make your experience more pleasant.
- Don't stress. Sharing your experiences with your child is a beautiful part of parenthood, and if you forget anything you can always buy it at your destination.

Expert Tips Before You Leave Home

- Pack a stroller frame for your car seat (for younger babies) or an umbrella stroller for older babies and toddlers, as it can be easier to help your child through the airport and the stroller can be checked at the gate. Your toddler's little legs may get tired, and your arms certainly will if you try to hold your carry-on luggage and your car seat at the same time.

- Pack a change of clothes for your baby or toddler just in case.
- Check in online before your leave, and if your airline has an app for your phone, make it available from your home screen for quick access during check-in.
- Put your identification card, and that of any family member traveling with you, in an easily accessible bag or purse so all hands can help your family get through the check-in and security process.
- Use uniquely colored luggage, or place a unique luggage tag on your bag, so it can be easily identified as it comes off the luggage carousel.
- If you're making hotel reservations, ask staff for a refrigerator (for pumped breast milk) or a portable crib, as many hotels offer these free of charge to travelers with babies or toddlers.
- For your 1- to 2-year-old, pack a "toddler bag," which has new games, books, toys, and snacks saved for the flight.

Expert Tips at the Airport
- If you're bringing pumped breast milk or pre-prepared formula with you, keep it in a side pocket as you move

through security, as it will likely need to be screened separately, and you'll want to be able to pull it out easily. This secondary screening process can take extra time, so get there early. One nice side note is that airlines do not specify a particular ounce limit for breast milk or formula, as you are allowed to bring as much as you need for your baby during the trip.

- Get to the gate as early as possible, as many airlines allow people requiring special assistance (including babies) to board before anyone else.
- If you have 2 adults, assign one to navigate the aisle and the seat with your child and the other to find overhead luggage room and to manage carry-on luggage.
- For babies younger than 2 months, remember that many viruses in crowded airports or planes can give them a fever and require medical attention, so be sure to keep their car seat covered as much as possible.
- Babies 2 to 12 months often do better with flying, as they nap during large portions of the day, feed often and more predictably (which is great for keeping ears clear during takeoffs and landings), and have protection against germs such as flu (if older than 6 months) and pneumonia if fully vaccinated.
- Giving your baby something to suck on, such as a pacifier or a bottle, can help takeoff and landing discomfort, as it may help his ears "pop" as the pressure changes.

- For a toddler 12 to 24 months, pull out your toddler bag to entertain him with special toys, games, books, stuffed animals, and healthy snacks. Take out one toy at a time so if your child gets bored with one, a new toy may seem exciting and entertain him for longer periods.

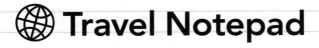 # Travel Notepad

Child's Name:

Important Travel Information:

Must-Bring Items:

☐

☐

☐

☐

☐

Other:

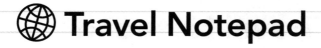 **Travel Notepad**

Child's Name:

Important Travel Information:

Must-Bring Items:

☐

☐

☐

☐

☐

Other:

RECOMMENDED WEB SITES

We recommend many Web sites to our patients and are fond of those under the watchful eye of the American Academy of Pediatrics (AAP).

The American Board of Pediatrics (www.abp.org). This Web site offers the ability to search the board certification status of doctors in your area.

HealthyChildren.org (www.healthychildren.org). This is the official AAP Web site of trusted content dedicated to parents. Current pediatric articles, news, and advice are available here. HealthyChildren.org also has a fantastic symptom checker, on which you can obtain advice based on your child's specific symptoms. You can download a version of the KidsDoc app onto your Android or Apple mobile device.

shopAAP (shop.aap.org/for-parents). Here you can purchase books recommended and published by the AAP.

Other helpful sites outside of the AAP include

Consumer Product Safety Division (www.cpsc.gov/en/recalls). This Web site features a comprehensive and current list of US product recalls.

Centers for Disease Control and Prevention Travelers' Health (http://wwwnc.cdc.gov/travel). This is the authority for information related to international travel, including diseases that may be widespread in a region and special immunizations or medications that may be recommended for travel to less developed countries.

Federal Aviation Administration Child Safety (www.faa.gov/passengers/fly_children). This Web site includes information about child safety with air travel, as well as tips about Child Restraint Systems and advice for travel with children with special needs.

SafeCar.gov (www.safercar.gov/parents/CarSeats.htm). Helpful advice can be found here about car seat use guidelines, installation, and ratings.

INDEX

Page numbers in *italic* denote figures.